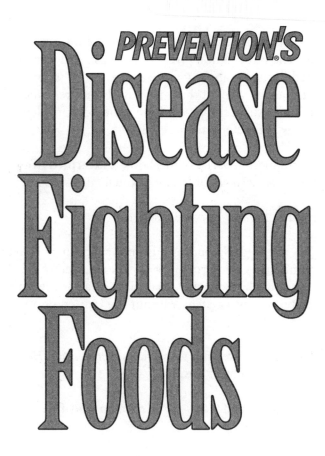

# PREVENTION'S
# Disease Fighting Foods

By the Editors of

**PREVENTION**™
**Health Books**

Rodale Press, Inc.
Emmaus, Pennsylvania

**Notice**
This book is intended as a reference volume only, not as a medical manual. The information given here is designed to help you make informed decisions about your health. It is not intended as a substitute for any treatment that may have been prescribed by your doctor. If you suspect that you have a medical problem, we urge you to seek competent medical help.

The information in part 2 of this book is excerpted from *Prevention's New Foods for Healing* (Rodale Press, 1998).

┌─────────── OUR PURPOSE ───────────┐
*"We inspire and enable people to improve*
*their lives and the world around them."*

# Contents

# Guide to Conditions

If you are interested in knowing about a specific health problem, you can use this guide to find the information you need. Simply look up the ailment, then turn to the page numbers listed to learn more about the foods that can prevent or treat it.

# L

**Low birthweight**
fish, 66, 68–69

**Lung ailments**
squash, 152

**Lung cancer**
carrots, 50, 51
garlic, 75
greens, 82
pumpkin, 133
tomatoes, 162

# M

**Macular degeneration**
apricots, 24
carrots, 50
greens, 83
pumpkin, 133
sea vegetables, 141

**Memory problems**
pears, 120

**Menopause**
soy foods, 147–48

**Migraines**
ginger, 78

**Motion sickness**
ginger, 77–78

# N

**Nasal congestion**
chili peppers, 57–58

# O

**Obesity**
*See* Overweight

**Osteoporosis**
broccoli, 42
milk, 94–95
pears, 120
pineapple, 124

**Ovarian cancer**
milk, 95

**Overweight**
broccoli, 43
figs, 64–65
water, 166

# P

**Polyps, colon**
asparagus, 27
melons, 91

**Prostate cancer**
broccoli, 42
brussels sprouts, 45
cabbage, 47
cauliflower, 54
soy foods, 37, 149
tomatoes, 161–62

# R

**Rectal cancer**
milk, 95
tomatoes, 162

**Respiratory diseases**
pumpkin, 133
squash, 152

# The
# Healing
# Powers
# of Nutrition

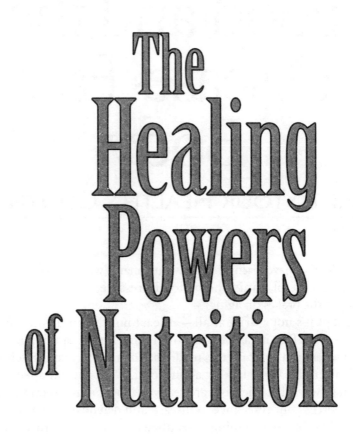

# Food and the Disease-Free Body

## EAT TO YOUR HEALTH'S CONTENT

Scientists have discovered a revolutionary "wonder drug" that can crush cholesterol, banish high blood pressure, combat cancer, and even put the brakes on aging.

Except it's not a drug at all—at least not the kind you buy in a drugstore. In fact, it has healing powers that no pill can duplicate.

So where can you find this medicinal marvel? Try your kitchen.

That's right: We're talking about food. What you eat affects your health in ways that scientists are really just beginning to understand. It reinforces your resistance to disease and defends against scores of medical problems, including heart disease, cancer, and stroke, the top three causes of death in the United States.

"When you sit down to a meal, you are dosing yourself with huge quantities of substances that will determine what's coursing through your body for the rest of the day," says Neal Barnard, M.D., president of the Physicians Committee for Responsible Medicine in Washington, D.C., and author of *Food for Life* and other books on the healing properties of foods. "Most people don't think of food as medication, but in reality, it is the single biggest medication that we're exposed to."

### FROM REJECTED TO RESPECTED

This represents quite a shift in philosophy for the mainstream medical community, which for years expressed skepticism about any suggested link between food and health. Until recently, few doctors received any formal training in basic nutrition.

"We're so busy learning how to fix broken arms, deliver babies, and do all of those 'doctor' things in medical school that we consider nutrition to be boring," says Michael A. Klaper, M.D., a nutritional medicine specialist in Pompano Beach, Florida, and director of the Institute of Nutritional Education and Research, an organization based in Manhattan Beach, California, that teaches doctors about nutrition and its relationship to disease. "But after we get into practice, we spend most of the day treating people with diseases that have huge nutritional components that have long been essentially ignored." Indeed, studies have implicated poor eating habits in a whole spectrum of ailments that ranges from acne to arthritis, from hair loss to hearing loss, from premenstrual syndrome to postnasal drip.

But after decades of depending on drugs to cure such ills, folks have become a lot more savvy about nutrition. They want to know what role it plays in their health and what foods might help make them better, Dr. Klaper notes. This, in turn, has forced the medical community to rethink its own attitude toward and approach to nutrition. Doctor and patient alike are at last realizing what a century ago was accepted as fact: Food is strong medicine.

## Mother (Nature) Knows Best

For thousands of years, folks around the world have used food to heal the sick and keep the healthy well. Archeological findings show that the ancient Sumerians, Assyrians, Akkadians, and Babylonians prized certain foods, herbs, and spices for their medicinal value. Ancient Egyptians treated asthma with figs, grapes, and even beer, and they touted garlic for curing infection and other conditions. And practitioners of Asian folk medicine have been "prescribing" celery since 200 B.C. as a remedy for high blood pressure.

Even the United States has a tradition of using food as medicine. Prior to the twentieth century, we were primarily a nation of small farms. Back then, people ate what they grew—mainly healthful "whole" foods such as grains, fruits, and vegetables. And since they didn't have antibiotics and other medications, their gardens served as medicine chests and their kitchens acted as pharmacies.

The Industrial Revolution changed everything, including our way of eating and our attitude toward food. The typical diet shifted from low-fat, high-fiber plant foods to high-fat, low-fiber animal foods.

# Straight from the Source

No one food can cover all your nutritional bases. That's why most experts stress a well-balanced, varied diet that features lots of high-fiber, low-fat foods such as fruits, vegetables, and whole grains.

Indeed, research has linked dietary diversity to a longer life span. In a study of 10,337 people, those with the most monotonous diets also had the highest mortality rates. Usually these folks ran low on fruits and vegetables. "It helps to choose foods from all food groups every day," concludes the study leader, Ashima K. Kant, Ph.D., professor of nutrition at Queens College of City University of New York.

Okay, we know what you're thinking: "Why can't I just take a supplement every day and be done with it?" Supplements are great if you're eating right but still coming up short on certain nutrients. But as their name suggests, they're intended as additions to a healthy diet, not as replacements for a poor one.

Only foods can supply you with carbohydrates, protein, and fiber, which your body needs just as much as vitamin and minerals to function properly. And only foods contain phytochemicals, little-known chemical compounds that scientists believe can protect against serious health problems such as heart disease and cancer, says Martha L. Rew, R.D., associate clinical professor of nutrition at Texas Woman's University in Denton.

What's more, research has yet to conclusively prove that vitamins and minerals from pills work just as well in the body as vitamins and minerals from foods. One thing is certain, though: It's quite easy to overdo supplements, possibly with serious consequences to your health. Besides, eating foods is a whole lot more pleasurable than just swallowing supplements. Foods have sensory appeal, offering an intoxicating array of aromas, textures, and flavors. Supplements are...well, pills, which means taking one is about as stimulating as popping an aspirin.

The bottom line: Look to foods first to get all the nutrients your body needs. Then maybe—*maybe*—opt for supplements to make up the difference between your daily dietary intake and your actual vitamin and mineral requirements.

"This contributed to many of the health problems we see today," Dr. Klaper says. "For instance, people rarely got cancer back then. And the first heart attack was documented in 1908, in the *Journal of the American Medical Association*."

After World War II, food's status as a remedy slowly eroded as we became enamored with a new breed of healing heroes. "We started relying on antibiotics and other so-called wonder drugs and paid less attention to food as medicine," explains Earl Mindell, R.Ph., Ph.D., professor of nutrition at Pacific Western University in Los Angeles and author of *Earl Mindell's Food as Medicine* and other books on nutrition. By the 1950s, food was simply something to make meals from— fuel for the body, nothing more.

These days, of course, the pendulum is swinging back. Scientists continue to uncover evidence of the pivotal role that food plays in our physical and emotional health. Based on what they've found so far, food has even greater healing powers than we realized.

## 25 Reasons to Eat Right

Of course, scientists have just scratched the surface in understanding the relationship between food and health. What they've turned up so far is quite impressive. Here's just a sampling of what eating right can do for you.

**Hinder heart disease.** Heart disease ranks as the number one cause of death in the United States. Many experts attribute this dubious distinction to a much-too-high intake of dietary fat. But they also believe that foods such as olive oil, soy, garlic, and grape juice can cut your odds of developing heart disease by nearly 25 percent.

**Clobber high cholesterol.** Too much cholesterol floating around in your bloodstream can plug up your arteries and set the stage for a heart attack, explains Penny Kris-Etherton, R.D., Ph.D., professor of nutrition at Pennsylvania State University in University Park. You probably already know that a high-fat diet can send your cholesterol levels through the roof. But now there's evidence that certain foods, especially fiber-rich beans and pectin-rich fruits such as grapefruit, can help keep your cholesterol low and your arteries clear.

**Collar high blood pressure.** High blood pressure is another common precursor of heart attack. About one of every four Americans has it. A quartet of nutrients that you can easily get from foods— calcium, magnesium, potassium, and vitamin C—may be all you need to whip your blood pressure reading into shape.

**Combat cancer.** The typical high-fat, high-calorie American diet is believed to contribute to as many as 60 percent of cancer cases among women and 40 percent among men. But by cutting down on dietary fat and filling up on fruits, vegetables, and whole grains, women could reduce their risk of breast cancer by one-quarter, while men could reduce their risk of prostate cancer by one-sixth. "We know from large population studies that people who eat lots of produce, in particular, are less likely to develop cancer," says Susan Taylor Mayne, Ph.D., associate director of cancer prevention and control research at the Yale University Cancer Center. "Fruits and vegetables contain compounds that in laboratory studies appear to block or suppress cancer growth."

**Stave off stroke.** Both high cholesterol and high blood pressure can dramatically increase your odds of suffering a stroke. Whether you have one or both of these risk factors, your first step in stroke prevention is to get them under control. You may be able to put even more distance between you and stroke by sprucing up your diet with fruits and vegetables. Produce has nutrients, including the B vitamin folate, that can protect against the arterial damage that leads to stroke.

**Derail diabetes.** Diet has a part to play in both the prevention and treatment of diabetes. In fact, if you have Type II (non-insulin-dependent) diabetes, you may very well be able to manage it simply by eating right and exercising regularly. And if you have Type I (insulin-dependent) diabetes, there's good news from the nutrition front for you, too: Preliminary research has suggested that consuming a diet rich in olive oil can reduce a person's need for insulin by 13 percent.

**Beef up your bones.** As many as one in two women and one in five men will experience an osteoporosis-related fracture sometime in their lives. You can cut your own risk in half just by making sure that you're getting enough bone-building calcium in your diet.

**Waylay weight gain.** This one could probably go without saying: A low-fat, low-calorie eating plan that includes lots of grains and produce is your best bet for saying bye-bye to extra baggage. And you have a very good reason to do so because overweight has been linked to serious health problems such as heart disease and cancer.

**Turn back the clock.** Many of the physical changes that occur as you get older—sagging skin, poor muscle tone, and reduced immunity, for example—can be traced to cellular damage from renegade molecules called free radicals. Neutralize these free radicals, the theory goes, and you can fend off the effects of aging. That's where the antioxidants—vitamins C and E and beta-carotene—come in. By eating foods rich in these nutrients, you can help slow the aging process and protect yourself against age-related disease.

**Enhance immunity.** Your body needs food to keep your immune system in good working order. It uses nutrients as raw material to manufacture and repair cells, which in turn improves your resistance to disease.

**Banish fatigue.** Complex carbohydrates such as whole grains, beans, and vegetables help keep your energy level on an even keel.They also supply the nutrients your body needs most when it's run-down.

**Short-circuit stress.** While research so far has yet to produce any definitive findings, many experts believe that prolonged stress depletes your body's supplies of key nutrients such as calcium and zinc. In stressful times, you really need to go the extra mile to feed your body properly, but it's worth the effort. There's also preliminary evidence that vitamin C can help protect your body against the effects of stress.

**Boost your brainpower.** You can turbocharge your alertness, concentration, and memory by munching on a bit of low-fat protein. What does protein have to do with cognitive skills? It supports the production of neurotransmitters that keep you mentally sharp.

**Safeguard reproductive health.** Like every other system in your body, your reproductive system depends on good nutrition to function properly. Researchers suspect that several aspects of reproduction, from sex drive to fertility, have a nutritional component.

**Tame premenstrual symptoms.** Women who experience premenstrual syndrome may find some relief with the help of vitamin $B_6$ and calcium. Both nutrients have shown potential for easing the irritability, insomnia, bloating, headache, edginess, constipation, fatigue, and breast tenderness that often precede monthly periods.

**Benefit baby.** If you're a woman who's planning to become pregnant, you can give your baby a healthy start by making sure that all your nutrient bases are covered. First and foremost, that means getting enough folate in your diet. This B vitamin appears to foster fetal development and protect against birth defects. Proper nutrition is also crucial if you plan to breastfeed.

**Master menopause.** Women in Japan experience fewer menopausal symptoms than women in the United States. And now researchers think they know why: because Japanese cuisine relies heavily on soy foods. Soy foods contain phytoestrogens, plant compounds that act much like the female hormone estrogen in the body. A dwindling supply of estrogen is what triggers menopause in the first place.

**Save your skin.** Eating healthfully can help prevent acne, canker sores, hives, and other minor skin eruptions. There's evidence, too, that chowing down on lots of fruits and vegetables can make you less likely to develop skin cancer.

**Spare your vision.** Macular degeneration is the leading cause of vision loss among older adults. But you can protect your eyes from this insidious disease—starting now—by eating plenty of leafy greens. Spinach, collard greens, and other verdant vegetables contain carotenoids, which at least one study has linked to a 43 percent reduction in risk of macular degeneration.

**Mollify migraine.** By one estimate, as many as one in five migraine attacks is provoked by something you've eaten. Experts believe that you can reduce the frequency and severity of migraines just by making changes in your diet, which means trading processed foods for whole, natural alternatives, especially grains and vegetables.

**Curb kidney stones.** An estimated 10 to 20 percent of men and 5 to 10 percent of women pass a kidney stone sometime in their lives. To avoid being one of them, your best bet is to lighten up on your salt intake—and drink lots and lots of water, of course.

**Derail digestive distress.** It should come as no surprise that a whole host of digestive ailments, from constipation to gallstones to irritable bowel syndrome, have a dietary component. Certain foods have a knack for tying your gut in knots. But others can ease your discomfort and keep the digestive process running smoothly.

**Override anemia.** Anemia, a condition that's usually characterized by extreme fatigue, results from a shortage of iron in the blood. It's especially widespread among women, according to Susan M. Lark, M.D., a physician in Los Altos, California, and author of *Chronic Fatigue and Tiredness*. The good news is that you can replenish your iron stores by eating foods that are rich in the mineral, such as lean meats and kidney beans.

**Ease arthritis.** It's controversial, but some experts believe that fish can help minimize arthritis pain. Many species supply healthy doses of omega-3 fatty acids, which can help keep your joints well-oiled and pain-free. Other studies suggest that high intakes of vitamins C and D can produce a threefold reduction in the progression of osteoarthritis, the most common form of arthritis.

**Protect your pearly whites.** Calcium, your body's main bone-builder, also plays a role in helping your teeth to stay healthy and strong. Vitamin C and folate also chip in, feeding the structures that support the teeth and helping to ward off infection.

# Healthy Eating Strategies

## FEED YOUR BODY RIGHT

Certain foods can fight disease and make you well. And likewise, a healthy, balanced diet can keep you from getting sick in the first place.

Of course, this begs the question, Just what is a healthy, balanced diet?

Truth be told, it's not always easy to know. While we have access to more nutrition information now than ever before, much of what we read or hear today contradicts what we read or heard yesterday—and what we'll be reading or hearing a week, a month, or a year from now. In fact, according to one survey, two-thirds of Americans say that they're confused by news reports telling them which foods they should avoid.

If this describes you, don't let frustration or disillusionment discourage you from your efforts to eat right. It's true that scientists will continue to make breakthrough discoveries that shoot holes in previous breakthrough discoveries. But it's also true that some nutrition principles have held up under scientific scrutiny, at least so far. You should use these can't-go-wrong rules as the foundation for building your own healthy eating habits.

What follows is an overview of the basics of good nutrition, along with some practical advice for incorporating them into your lifestyle. If you're in need of motivation, just remember that even modest changes in your eating habits can substantially reduce your risk of developing an array of illnesses. And let's be honest: Switching from potato chips to carrots is an insignificant price to pay for a lifetime of good health.

## Pyramid Power

The road to proper nutrition begins at the pyramid—that is, the Food Guide Pyramid. You've probably seen it: a four-tier triangle that outlines which foods you should eat every day, and in what amounts, to give your body the nutrients it needs to efficiently perform even the most routine tasks. It has changed the way many of us look at our dinner plates.

Unlike its predecessor, the Four Food Groups, the pyramid gives grains, fruits, and vegetables top priority, since they offer the most nutrients for the lowest amount of fat. Meats and dairy products, meanwhile, have been downgraded from mainstays to virtual blips.

According to the U.S. Department of Agriculture, which developed the Food Guide Pyramid, this new nutrition icon sets more realistic standards for what people should be eating. It also encourages the consumption of a variety of foods—a balanced, everything-in-moderation approach to eating—while keeping a lid on fat and calories.

The pyramid consists of these six food groups. (*Note:* The recommendations for each food group include a range of servings. The low number in the range applies to someone who requires just 1,600 calories a day, most likely a sedentary woman. The high number, on the other hand, is for someone who eats 2,800 calories a day, most likely an active man. You need to gauge your own activity level and set your daily serving requirements accordingly.)

**Grains.** Grain-based foods—breads, cereals, rice, and pasta—make up the foundation of the pyramid. They supply a multitude of nutrients, including complex carbohydrates, vitamins, minerals, and fiber. According to the pyramid, you should aim for 6 to 11 servings of grains per day, with a serving being equal to one slice of bread, 1 ounce of cold cereal, or $^1/_2$ cup of cooked cereal, rice, or pasta.

**Vegetables.** The pyramid recommends three to five servings a day of veggies, which offer healthy doses of vitamins, minerals, and fiber. A serving consists of 1 cup of raw leafy vegetables, $^1/_2$ cup of chopped cooked or raw vegetables, or $^3/_4$ cup of vegetable juice.

**Fruits.** Like vegetables, fruits have abundant supplies of vitamins, minerals, and fiber. Try to consume two to four servings a day. A medium apple, banana, or orange; $^1/_2$ cup of chopped, cooked, or canned fruit; or $^3/_4$ cup of fruit juice all constitute a serving.

**Dairy products.** Milk, yogurt, cheese, and other foods in this group are outstanding sources of protein and calcium. You should eat two to three servings a day, with a serving defined as 1 cup of milk or yogurt, $1^1/_2$ ounces of "natural" cheese, or 2 ounces of processed cheese.

**Meats.** Actually, you could call this group meats-plus, since it also includes poultry, fish, dried beans, eggs, and nuts. These foods provide generous amounts of protein as well as the minerals zinc and iron. The pyramid recommends two to three servings from this group every day. A serving equals 2 to 3 ounces of cooked lean meat, poultry, or fish (an amount that's about the size of your palm); $^1/_2$ cup of cooked dried beans; one egg; or 2 tablespoons of peanut butter.

**Fats, oils, and sweets.** The pyramid has just two words for this group: "Use sparingly." Enough said.

## BEYOND THE BASICS

The Food Guide Pyramid sets very solid ground rules for good nutrition. Shape your diet around the pyramid's serving suggestions and you ensure that you're getting the right mix of nutrients to keep your body properly fueled.

To bolster your body's resistance to disease, however, you need to look past the pyramid. The following strategies will help strengthen your diet's health-promoting potential.

**Eschew the fat.** The human body uses dietary fat to transport vitamins, protect vital organs, maintain body temperature, and perform other essential tasks. Unfortunately, most of us consume a lot more of the stuff than our bodies actually need. In excess, dietary fat contributes to heart disease, cancer, diabetes, and obesity. Many experts suggest limiting your fat intake to 30 percent of calories, while some suggest cutting back even more, to 25 percent of calories.

**Count on carbs.** There's a reason that complex-carbohydrate foods such as grains, fruits, and vegetables make up the bottom two tiers of the Food Guide Pyramid. Complex carbohydrates are your body's fuel of choice because they easily break down into a form that your body uses to keep all its systems running smoothly and efficiently. Experts recommend consuming 55 to 60 percent of your calories as carbohydrates.

**Favor fiber.** Coincidentally, when you eat carbohydrate-rich foods, you're also getting a good dose of fiber. Research has shown that fiber helps improve digestion, lower blood cholesterol, and reduce your odds of developing heart disease and cancer. The Daily Value for fiber is 25 grams.

**Get wet.** More than 50 percent of your body is water. Over the course of a day, you lose a lot of $H_2O$ through urine, sweat, and respiration. That's why experts advise adults to drink about a quart of water for every 1,000 calories in their diets. So if you eat 2,000 calories a day, you should wash them down with 2 quarts of water (that's 64 ounces, or eight 8-ounce glasses a day). Of course, your fluid needs increase when you exercise and when the weather is hot.

**Know your limits.** When it comes to sugar, salt, and alcohol, the less you consume, the better. Refined sugar, the stuff in candy and packaged snacks, wreaks havoc on your metabolism in exchange for zero nutrition benefits. Too much salt can contribute to high blood pressure. And excessive alcohol consumption increases your risk of cancer and interferes with nutrient absorption.

**Shore up with supplements.** You should get most of your vitamins and minerals from foods. One reason is that foods contain compounds called phytochemicals, little-known "supernutrients" that possess tremendous disease-fighting powers. You won't find these compounds in pills—at least, not yet.

Still, the law of nutrition reality says that we don't always eat as we should. When you know that your diet is coming up short, a multivitamin can pick up the slack. Just remember that a supplement is not a more-is-better thing. Some vitamins and minerals are toxic in high doses.

Good nutrition starts long before you take a seat at the dinner table and pick up your knife and fork. "To eat healthy, you must buy healthy," notes Bonnie Tandy Leblang, R.D., author of the nationally syndicated column "Supermarket Sampler" and six cookbooks, including *Grains, Rice, and Beans.* "Smart supermarket strategies are the key to eating well at home."

Of course, it would be nice to think that the supermarket you frequent shares your concerns about good nutrition. To some extent, it probably does. Many chain stores have instituted consumer education programs, posting signs and distributing pamphlets that detail the nutritional values of specific items.

Still, their bottom line is...well, the bottom line. They want you to spend—and to leave the store with more items than the two or three you originally planned to buy. And so they invest literally billions of dollars in dizzying, dazzling displays designed to make the most of every selling opportunity. You can resist such temptations and stay true to your healthy eating habits by learning these grocery guidelines.

**Learn label lingo.** Label reading has become a necessary skill for nutrition-conscious shoppers. Compared with labels of five years ago, the ones we see these days present a veritable *Encyclopaedia Britannica* of nutrition information. An ingredients list and a Nutrition Facts chart graces nearly every packaged food. They tell you not only what a particular product is made from but also how much of certain nutrients it contains. That way, you can decide whether that product has a place in your healthy diet.

**Cruise the perimeter.** A shopping list is your most important navigational tool for getting around the supermarket, experts agree. But if you don't have one to go by, try to stay in the store's outside aisles as much as you can. "This is where you'll find the fresh foods, especially produce," says Michele Tuttle, R.D., director of consumer affairs for the Food Marketing Institute in Washington, D.C.

**See the "lite" in the dairy case.** The dairy case stocks the cream of the calcium crop. Milk, yogurt, and cheese all weigh in with generous amounts of the mineral. Unfortunately, the regular varieties of these foods also have generous amounts of fat. Select leaner alternatives when you can, such as skim or 1% low-fat milk and nonfat or low-fat yogurt. Likewise, the healthiest choices in cheese are made from skim or low-fat milk and are not highly processed.

**Be Selective with meats.** There are three grades, or qualities, of beef sold in most supermarkets. Prime cuts have the most fat, Select cuts have the least, and Choice cuts fall somewhere in between. You want to look for cuts stamped Select. The less marbling a piece of meat has, the leaner it is. Sure, you can trim the fat yourself, but you save money if you buy it already trimmed. (Prime cuts are actually more expensive than Select cuts because they have more fat.)

**Stock up on seafood.** Tucked somewhere between the dairy case and the meat counter is the seafood display. Don't pass it by. With the exception of anchovies, almost any fish or shellfish that you can think of has nutritional benefit. Some, like Atlantic herring, canned salmon, fresh tuna, and Atlantic mackerel, are rich in omega-3 fatty acids. There's medical evidence that omega-3's can reduce heart-unhealthy triglycerides, inhibit the growth of breast cancer cells, and even prevent gallstones.

Some seafood does contain cholesterol, but it's not the type that raises the level of cholesterol in your blood. Shellfish are a good example: They don't have a lot of saturated fat, so the cholesterol they supply isn't a big concern. Do steer clear of prepared seafood salads, though; they're bound to be loaded with fat.

**Don't bypass beans.** Swing into the inside supermarket aisles to stock up on beans and other legumes. They pack a nutritional one-two

# How Much Do You Need?

Take a look at the nutrition information on any packaged food and you'll see the abbreviation DV. It stands for Daily Value, a federal government guideline for how much of a certain nutrient you should be getting each day. There are Daily Values established for 19 vitamins and minerals as well as for carbohydrates, protein, fat, and fiber.

The "Percent Daily Value" on a food's label shows how that food helps you meet your daily nutrient needs. The percentages are calculated for a 2,000-calorie-a-day diet. If you're eating fewer calories than that, as many women do, keep in mind that you'll be getting smaller amounts of the nutrients as well.

To quickly assess a food's nutritional value, use these rules of thumb: For total fat, cholesterol, and sodium, each percent Daily Value should not exceed 100 percent—and the lower, the better. For fiber, vitamins A and C, calcium, and iron, higher amounts are ideal. (In general, food labels list only these four vitamins and minerals because people tend to not get enough of them.)

Keep in mind that while the DVs maintain the nutritional status quo for healthy people, some experts believe that you must consume much higher amounts of certain nutrients to treat or prevent specific illnesses. "Generally, I'd say that vitamins and minerals in amounts well above the DVs are safe for most people," says Gladys Block, Ph.D., professor of epidemiology and director of the public health nutrition program at the University of California, Berkeley.

punch of protein and fiber, and they're filling and versatile to boot.

And while you're there, check out the grain products. Brown rice, for instance, supplies notable amounts of fiber and the B vitamins $B_6$, niacin, and thiamin in exchange for no cholesterol and just a smidgen of fat. You may also want to try bulgur. It has even more fiber than rice with no cholesterol and practically no fat.

## THE HIGH-NUTRITION KITCHEN

Healthy cooking has long had a reputation as a time-consuming, costly, complicated venture. The truth is, it doesn't require exotic, hard-to-find ingredients or expensive, top-of-the-line equipment. For that matter, it doesn't require any special culinary skills: Even a novice can whip up nutritious, balanced meals quickly and easily. Here's what you need to know.

**Plan ahead.** The real trick of the healthy cooking trade, nutritionists agree, is to heed the Boy Scout motto and be prepared. "When you don't have a lot of time, you're more likely to make unhealthy food choices," says Suzanne Havala, R.D., a nutritionist in Charlotte, North Carolina, and author of *Simple, Low-Fat, and Vegetarian.* "It helps to take a little time each week to preplan your meals."

You may want to try setting aside an hour or so each weekend to lay out a menu for the week ahead, suggests Judith Gilliard, author of *The Guiltless Gourmet* and other cookbooks. Besides making life easier during the week, when your time and energy are at a premium, a menu helps ensure that you're eating a balanced diet with the right amounts of the right foods and not shortchanging yourself nutrition-wise.

**Do the 'wave.** When it comes to healthy cooking, nothing beats microwaving. Besides saving time, it also saves nutrients, not to mention flavor. Steaming takes longer, but it also does a good job of preserving nutrients. The reason: The food is cooked over water rather than in it.

**Season with abandon.** While we once relied on fat and salt to give our foods taste, we now know that we need to cut back on this dietary dastardly duo for the sake of good nutrition—and good health. Herbs and spices more than fill this flavor void. And they do it while supplying just a smidgen of fat, sodium, and calories.

The following selections make an ideal seasoning starter kit that should cover many of your cooking needs. Besides being quite versatile, these herbs and spices offer so many important health benefits that they're almost too good to pass up.

| | |
|---|---|
| • Basil | • Horseradish |
| • Bay leaf | • Paprika |
| • Cinnamon | • Parsley |
| • Cloves | • Red pepper flakes |
| • Cumin | • Rosemary |
| • Garlic | • Turmeric |
| • Ginger | |

**Send in the substitutions.** A little culinary sleight of hand goes a long way in cutting the fat content of your favorite recipes and sparing them from mealtime extinction. By exchanging high-fat ingredients for leaner alternatives, you can keep on eating the foods you love. Here are some examples.

- In baked goods, replace $1/2$ cup of oil with $1/2$ cup of applesauce to save 109 grams of fat.
- In salad dressings, replace $1/2$ cup of oil with $1/2$ cup of unsweetened pineapple juice to save 109 grams of fat.
- In baked goods, replace $1/2$ cup of margarine or butter with $1/2$ cup of baby food prunes to save 92 grams of fat.
- In frostings, replace $1/2$ cup of margarine or butter with $1/2$ cup of marshmallow creme to save 92 grams of fat.
- In recipes that call for cream cheese, replace 8 ounces of cream cheese with 8 ounces of nonfat ricotta cheese to save 79 grams of fat.
- Replace one whole egg with two egg whites to save 5 grams of fat.

**Save your skin.** It's fine—in fact, it's preferable—to cook poultry with the skin on. The fat doesn't migrate from the skin into the meat. Even better, the skin helps the meat retain its moistness. Do, however, remove the skin before eating the poultry. This simple step slashes about 50 grams of fat off a typical 4-pound chicken.

## MEALS ON THE MOVE

While we still seem to prefer our own home cookin', our never-a-minute-to-spare lifestyles mean that we do a lot more eating out these days. We grab food when we can, where we can, be it breakfast from a convenience store, lunch from a fast-food chain, or a snack from a vending machine.

Obviously, eating away from home can easily compromise your healthy eating habits. On the other hand, it can expand your opportunities for satisfying your body's nutrient requirements. To maximize the nutrition benefits of your dining-out experience, heed this advice from the experts.

**Bank on breakfast.** Eating a morning meal gives your body a running start nutrition wise. "You are literally breaking a fast—your body hasn't had food for the past 8 to 12 hours," explains Elizabeth Somer, R.D., author of *Nutrition for Women* and *Food and Mood.* "If you skip breakfast, you may not rebuild your energy stores for the day."

Take advantage of the opportunity to squeeze in a couple of servings of fruit. Have a glass of orange juice as a breakfast "appetizer," then slice up a banana on your cereal.

**Pack your own snacks.** Turn your purse or briefcase into a portable vending machine that dispenses healthy snacks: cans of low-sodium tomato juice, mini-boxes of raisins, packs of whole-grain crackers, and bags of baby carrots. And don't forget to grab an apple to munch on during your commute home.

**Get servings on the side.** When you eat in a restaurant, order an extra side dish or two of vegetables. This will help ensure that you get enough fiber, vitamins, and minerals with your meal. Eat those veggies plain, though—no cream sauce, cheese, or butter.

**Make it plain.** Your lunch hour has shrunk to 20 minutes, and you have just enough time to grab something at the nearest fast-food drive-up window. What will it be?

Your best bet is to order the smallest burger on the menu, with ketchup and mustard, if you like, but without cheese or special sauce. Ask for extra lettuce and tomatoes. Then swing by the nearest convenience store for some fresh fruit and a pint of nonfat milk to complete the meal.

**Order nutrients by the slice.** Pizza as a health food? Well, think about it. Pizza has tomato sauce, and tomatoes are the top source of cancer-fighting lycopene. It has olive oil, a monounsaturated fat that can help give the old heave-ho to LDL cholesterol (the bad kind). For toppings, you can choose onions for heart-healthy flavonoids and broccoli for cancer-fighting carotenoids. Even oregano has some benefit: It's a potent antioxidant.

To keep your pizza healthy, request nonfat or low-fat cheese in half the usual amount or even less. Also, bypass high-fat extras such as pepperoni, sausage, and hamburger.

**Belly up to the (salad) bar.** Depending on what goes in it, a salad can be either a top-notch health food or a dietary disaster. To beef up your salad's nutritional profile, choose dark leafy greens such as romaine lettuce, kale, spinach, watercress, and arugula over iceberg lettuce. Then add your choice of the following toppings.

| | |
|---|---|
| • Beets | • Cucumbers |
| • Broccoli florets | • Mushrooms |
| • Carrots | • Peppers |
| • Cauliflower | • Red cabbage |
| • Celery | • Tomatoes |

Steer clear of the olives, bacon bits, chopped eggs, croutons, and chow mein noodles as well as premade, mayonnaise-based salads. If you must have dressing, choose a nonfat or low-fat variety. Rather than drizzling it over your salad, leave it on the side and lightly dip your fork in it before taking a bite. This method gives you better portion control.

# Foods That Heal

# Apples

## THEIR BENEFITS ARE SKIN-DEEP

It's really not surprising that apples have long been considered a symbol of good health and vitality. For one thing, you can keep them handy to eat anywhere, anytime, just by dropping one in your briefcase, backpack, or purse. To complete the package, they come ready-wrapped in their own protective but tasty skin, with all their tart sweetness wrapped within. It's almost as if the head designer said, "Apples are good, so I'll make them easy to eat."

Yet apples are more than just a wholesome snack. Studies suggest that eating apples can help reduce the risk of heart disease. In the laboratory, they have been shown to have stopping power against cancer cells. Evidence is still preliminary, but it appears that having an apple or two a day really can help keep the doctor away.

### IT'S ALL IN THE SKIN

Even though many people favor the flesh, much of an apple's healing power resides in the skin, which contains large amounts—about 4 milligrams—of a compound called quercetin. Like vitamin C and beta-carotene, this is an antioxidant compound that can help prevent harmful oxygen molecules from damaging individual cells. Over time, this can help prevent changes in the cells that can lead to cancer.

Even in the healing world of antioxidants, quercetin is thought to be exceptional. In one study, researchers in Finland compared the amount of various antioxidants in people's diets with their risk of heart disease over a 20-year period. Men who had the highest daily intake of quercetin and other antioxidants (their diets included about a quarter of an apple) had a 20 percent lower risk of heart disease than men who ate the least. The researchers concluded that quercetin was responsible for most of the study's good results.

In a study in the Netherlands, researchers found that men eating an apple a day (along with 2 tablespoons of onions and four cups of tea) had a 32 percent lower risk of heart attack than those who ate fewer apples.

"So an apple a day is not a bad idea," says Lawrence H. Kushi, Sc.D., associate professor of public health, nutrition, and epidemiology at the University of Minnesota in Minneapolis.

Heart disease isn't the only major malady to feel quercetin's force. The compound has also shown clout against cancer. Laboratory studies show that it can inhibit the growth of tumors and also help prevent cancer cells from spreading.

"When you subject single cells to a carcinogen and then put in quercetin, you prevent mutation from occurring—you prevent the carcinogen from acting," says Dr. Kushi. "Quercetin is one of the things that apples are relatively high in."

## FIELDS OF FIBER

Recent discoveries aside, apples are perhaps best known for their fiber. They contain both soluble and insoluble fiber, including pectin. A 5-ounce apple with the skin has about 3 grams of fiber. "They're a good source," says Chang Lee, Ph.D., professor of food science and technology at Cornell University–New York State Agricultural Experimental Station in Geneva.

Insoluble fiber, found mostly in the skin, is the kind that we used to call roughage, which has long been recommended for relieving constipation. More is at stake, though, than just comfort. Studies show that a smoothly operating digestive tract can help prevent diverticulosis, a condition in which small pouches form in the large intestine, and also cancer of the colon. Plus, insoluble fiber is filling, which is why apples are such an excellent weight-control food.

The soluble fiber in apples, which is the same kind found in oat bran, acts differently from the insoluble kind. Rather than passing through the digestive tract more or less unchanged, soluble fiber forms a gel-like material in the digestive tract that helps lower cholesterol and, with it, the risk of heart disease and stroke.

One type of soluble fiber, called pectin, appears to reduce the amount of cholesterol produced in the liver, providing double protection. "Plus, pectin's ability to form a gel slows digestion, which slows the rise in blood sugar—so it's good for people with diabetes," says Joan Walsh, R.D., Ph.D., foods and nutritional instructor at San Joaquin Delta College in Stockton, California.

An average-size apple contains 0.7 gram of pectin, more than the amount in strawberries and bananas.

# Getting the Most

**Look for the brown.** "Some varieties of apple, like Granny Smith, are bred to be low in certain protective compounds because that's what makes apples brown when you peel them," says Mary Ellen Camire, Ph.D., associate professor and chair of the department of food science and human nutrition at the University of Maine in Orono. Look for varieties that brown easily to reap the most health benefits.

**Don't count on apple juice.** Although apple juice contains a little iron and potassium, it's no great shakes compared to the whole fruit. By the time apples wind up as juice, they've given up most of their fiber and quercetin.

Of course, if you're choosing between soda and apple juice, by all means choose the juice. But don't use it as a substitute for the real thing.

# Apricots

## A BOUNTY OF BETA-CAROTENE

At one time, Chinese brides nibbled on apricots to increase fertility. It sounds funny today, until you realize that these fruits are, in fact, high in a mineral needed for the production of sex hormones.

These days, of course, few people are likely to rely on apricots to influence family size. Yet this sweet, velvety fruit contains a variety of compounds that research shows can fight infections, blindness, and heart disease.

Most of apricots' health benefits are due to their copious and exceptionally diverse carotenoid content. Carotenoids are the pigments in plants that paint many of our favorite fruits and vegetables red, orange, and yellow and that in humans have a wide range of health-protecting properties. Researchers have identified at least 600 different carotenoids, with some of the most powerful, including beta-carotene, being found in apricots.

"Apricots are one of the best foods to look to for carotenoids," says Ritva Butrum, Ph.D., vice president for research at the American Institute for Cancer Research in Washington, D.C. "Not only are they one of the richest carotenoid foods in terms of quantity, but also they have a wide variety of carotenoids."

### FRUIT FOR THE HEART

The apricot's unique mix of healing compounds makes this food a powerful ally in fighting heart disease. Along with beta-carotene , apricots contain lycopene, and both compounds have been shown in studies to fight the process by which the dangerous low-density lipoprotein (LDL) form of cholesterol turns rancid in the bloodstream. This is important because when LDL goes bad, it's more likely to stick to artery walls.

"Lycopene is currently considered one of the strongest antioxidants we know about," says Frederick Khachik, Ph.D., research chemist at the Food Composition Laboratory at the U.S. Department of Agriculture in Beltsville, Maryland.

A 13-year study found that those with the highest intakes of carotenoids had a one-third lower risk of heart disease than those with the lowest intakes. In an 8-year study of 90,000 nurses, those with diets richest in carotenoids had a one-quarter lower risk.

Apricots are a good source of beta-carotene, with three fruits containing 2 milligrams, about 30 percent of the recommended daily amount. Experts still aren't sure how much lycopene there is in apricots or for that matter, how much lycopene you need for good health. However, since these fruits are rich in several other carotenoids, says Dr. Khachik, you can't go wrong adding more to your diet.

## GOOD FOR THE EYES

Even if you don't have the spinach-loving personality of Popeye, you can get lots of vitamin A by eating apricots. (The beta-carotene in apricots is converted to vitamin A in the body.) This nutrient helps to protect the eyes, and it turns out that the eyes need all the help that they can get.

Every time light passes through the eyes, it triggers the release of tissue-damaging free radicals. Left unchecked, these destructive oxygen molecules attack and damage the lenses of the eyes, possibly setting the stage for cataracts. Free radicals can also attack blood vessels supplying the central portion of the retina, called the macula. If the blood supply gets cut off, the result can be maculars degeneration, the leading cause of irreversible vision loss in older adults.

Vitamin A has been shown in studies to be a powerful antioxidant—that is, it helps block the effects of free radicals. A study of more than 50,000 nurses, for example, found that women who got the most vitamin A in their diets reduced their risk of getting cataracts by more than one-third. (That same vitamin A also helps the body fight colds and other respiratory infections .) Three apricots provide 2,769 international units of vitamin A, 55 percent of the Daily Value (DV).

While apricots don't provide nearly as much vitamin A as carrots or dark green, leafy vegetables such as spinach and collard greens, they do provide an easy-to-eat alternative for those who simply don't have a taste for spinach.

## Help from Fiber

It's almost impossible to exaggerate the benefits of getting enough fiber in your diet. High-fiber foods can help you lose weight, control high blood sugar, and lower cholesterol levels. They're also essential for keeping digestion regular.

So here's another reason to add apricots to your fruit bowl. Three fruits contain 3 grams of fiber, 12 percent of the DV. Better yet, that's at a minimal calorie cost—just 51 calories for all three. When you're eating apricots for fiber, however, be sure to eat the skin, which contains a substantial amount of the fruit's fiber.

# Getting the Most

**Eat them firm.** Even if you enjoy your fruit nice and soft, it's best to eat apricots while they're still slightly firm. Apricots contain the most nutrients when they're at their peak of ripeness; once they start getting soft, these compounds quickly begin to break down.

**Shop for color.** Unlike most fruits, apricots can be yellow or orange and still be ripe. Both colors are acceptable when you're trying to get the most healing benefits. However, apricots with green in them means that they were picked early and may never ripen, which also means that you lose out on much of their healing goodness.

**Store them carefully.** It's important to keep apricots cool to prevent them from getting overripe. Unless you're going to eat them within a day or two, it's best to store them in the fruit bin in the refrigerator, where they'll keep for about a week.

Here's another storage tip: Because apricots are such a soft, delicate fruit, they readily pick up flavors—from other fruit they're stored with, for example, or even from refrigerator smells. It's a good idea to store them in a paper or plastic bag.

# Asparagus
## SPEARS OF PROTECTION

Asparagus was extremely popular among the royal households of seventeenth-century France—not just for its fresh taste but also because the tender spears were thought to be a powerful aphrodisiac.

For asparagus aficionados—even those without amour on the brain—there's no more welcome sign of spring than those brilliant green tips poking up from winter's ground. It's a welcome sign for health as well, since asparagus contains compounds that can help fight birth defects, heart disease, and cancer.

### FILLED WITH FOLATE

One of the most critical medical breakthroughs of this century was the discovery that the incidence of brain and spinal cord birth defects (called neural tube defects) could be cut in half if women of childbearing age got 400 micrograms of folate a day.

Asparagus is richly endowed with folate, a B vitamin that is essential for helping cells regenerate. Five asparagus spears contain 110 micrograms of folate, about 28 percent of the Daily Value (DV).

If you're pregnant, however, you may want to take a double serving. While government guidelines recommend that women get 400 micrograms of folate a day, folate researcher Lynn B. Bailey, Ph.D., professor of nutrition at the University of Florida in Gainesville, suggests that the optimal level for pregnant women may be higher, "possibly as high as 600 micrograms," she says.

Not only is folate good for women in their childbearing years, it also fights heart disease in everyone. It appears that folate acts as a floodgate, controlling the amount of homocysteine (an amino acid) in the bloodstream. When folate levels drop, homocysteine levels rise, causing damage to the tender arteries supplying blood to the heart and brain.

For preventing heart disease, getting enough folate may be just as important as controlling cholesterol. Indeed, heart researchers say that if Americans would increase their intake of folate to 400 micrograms a day, the number of deaths caused by heart disease would drop by at least 13,500. Currently, only 12 percent of us are getting that much.

## PROTECTION AGAINST CANCER

As you've come to expect from all the green vegetables, asparagus offers powerful protection against cancer. It contains a number of compounds that essentially double-team cancer-causing substances before they do harm.

The first of these substances is folate. Studies reveal that people with the most folate in their blood are the ones least likely to develop colon cancer. They're also less likely to develop polyps, small intestinal growths that over time can lead to cancer. In addition, there's evidence that folate guards against cervical cancer, especially in women infected with human papillomavirus, the virus that causes genital warts.

The second protective compound in asparagus is glutathione. A small protein, glutathione is a powerful antioxidant. This means that it helps mop up free radicals, high-energy particles that, when left unchecked, ricochet wildly through the body, scarring and punching holes in cells, and doing the types of damage that can lead to cancer. In an analysis of 38 vegetables, freshly cooked asparagus ranked first for its glutathione content.

## TAKE THE E TRAIN

There's another reason to add more asparagus to your plate. It contains vitamin E, which can be very good for the heart. A study led by researchers at the University of Minnesota School of Public Health in Minneapolis found that getting as little as 10 international units of vitamin E a day can substantially reduce the risk of heart disease in women. Five asparagus spears have 0.4 international unit of vitamin E. That's about 1 percent of the DV.

"This is the first study to examine the effect of vitamin E from food instead of from supplements, and the results surprised even us," says Lawrence H. Kushi, Sc.D., associate professor of public health, nutrition, and epidemiology at the University of Minnesota in Minneapolis and the lead investigator of the study.

Obviously, you'd have to eat a lot of asparagus (119 spears, to be exact) to get the amount of vitamin E that proved most beneficial in the study. In fact, it's difficult to get large amounts of vitamin E from diet alone since it's most abundant in oils and nuts. That's why many doctors recommend taking vitamin E supplements.

Vitamin E does more than protect against heart disease. Research suggests that it may even help prevent Type II, or non-insulin-dependent, diabetes, both by protecting the pancreas (the organ that produces insulin) and by influencing how the body burns sugar. A study of 944 men ages 42 to 60 found that men with low levels of vitamin E had nearly four times the risk of developing this disease.

# Getting the Most

**Store it carefully.** Folate is destroyed by exposure to air, heat, or light; so you need to store asparagus carefully, says Gertrude Armbruster, R.D., Ph.D., director of the dietetic program at Cornell University in Ithaca, New York. She recommends storing it away from light in the back of the refrigerator or in a produce drawer. It's also a good idea to protect it from air by keeping it well-wrapped in plastic, she says.

**Cook it gently.** Asparagus is a tender vegetable, and vigorous boiling isn't necessary. What's more, boiling leaches out many of the beneficial nutrients, says Dr. Armbruster. "Microwaving asparagus definitely destroys fewer nutrients than does boiling or even steaming," she says.

**Stand it upright.** Since most of asparagus's nutrients are in the tip, it's better to cook it upright in a tall container rather than piling it at the bottom of a baking dish, Dr. Armbruster says. Add a few inches of water to the pot, cover with a lid, and bring to a simmer. Keeping the tips out of the water will not only preserve nutrients but will also help the stalks cook evenly and more quickly.

# Avocados

## No Longer Forbidden Fruit

Ounce for ounce, the humble avocado packs more calories than almost any other fruit on the planet: 731. It also has the dubious distinction of being one of the few fruits with a measurable fat content, with up to 30 grams each. That's half the daily recommended amount for an average adult.

You wouldn't think that a food that's so fattening could be good for you. But that's the word from dietitians, who say that adding a little avocado to your diet every day could actually improve your health.

Avocados are great sources of folate and potassium. They also contain high amounts of fiber and monounsaturated fat, both of which are good news for people who are concerned with diabetes or heart health.

### Part of a Diabetes Diet

People with diabetes have traditionally been told to eat more carbohydrates and cut back on fat. Overall that's good advice, but it's not necessarily the best advice for everyone.

Doctors have discovered that when some people who have diabetes eat a lot of carbohydrates, they tend to develop high levels of triglycerides, a type of blood fats that may contribute to heart disease. Surprisingly, when people replace some of those carbohydrates with fat, particularly the kind of fat found in avocados, the dangerous fats in the bloodstream tend to decline.

Avocados are a rich source of monounsaturated fats, particularly a kind called oleic acid. "We've found that these monounsaturated fats improve fat levels in the body and help control diabetes," says Abhimanyu Garg, M.D., associate professor of internal medicine and clinical nutrition at the University of Texas Southwestern Medical Center at Dallas.

In one study, scientists in Mexico put 16 women with diabetes on a relatively high-fat diet, with about 40 percent of calories coming from fat. Most of the fat came from avocados. The result was a 20 percent drop in triglycerides. Women on a higher-carbohydrate plan, by contrast, had only a 7 percent drop in triglycerides.

"What's nice about avocados is that they provide a lot of monounsaturated fats," adds Dr. Garg. Someone on a 2,000-calorie-a-day diet, for example, might be advised to eat 33 grams of fat. "You can get about 20 grams from just one avocado," he says.

## Help for High Cholesterol

People with diabetes aren't the only ones who benefit from eating a little more avocado. The oleic acid in avocados can also help people lower their cholesterol.

In small study from Mexico, where guacamole is considered almost a food group, researchers compared the effects of two low-fat diets. The diets were the same except that one included avocados. While both lowered levels of dangerous, low-density lipoprotein cholesterol, the avocado diet raised levels of healthful high-density lipoprotein cholesterol while slightly lowering triglycerides.

Another way in which avocados help lower cholesterol is by adding healthful amounts of fiber to the diet, adds Dr. Garg. Fiber adds bulk to the stool, causing it, and the cholesterol it contains, to be excreted from the body more quickly. One avocado packs more fiber than a bran muffin—10 grams, 40 percent of the Daily Value (DV).

By knocking down cholesterol, a high-fiber diet also helps prevent high blood pressure and heart disease. It can also reduce the risk of certain cancers, particularly colon cancer.

## More Help for Your Heart

Although bananas are generally the stars of the potassium spotlight, avocados also pack a big potassium punch. Half an avocado provides 548 milligrams of potassium, 16 percent of the DV. That's 15 percent more than you'd get in a medium banana.

Studies show that people who eat diets high in potassium-rich foods like avocados have a markedly lower risk of high blood pressure and related diseases like heart attack and stroke.

"You can never get too much potassium," says David B. Young, Ph.D., professor of physiology and biophysics at the University of Mississippi Medical Center in Jackson. Even small additions can make big differences, he says. Avocados are also a good source of magnesium, another mineral that's known for helping to keep blood pressure in the safety zone. Half an avocado provides about 35 milligrams of magnesium, 9 percent of the DV.

## A FORTUNE IN FOLATE

Avocados may be one of the perfect foods when you're eating for two, particularly when it comes to getting enough folate, a nutrient that helps prevent life-threatening birth defects of the brain and spine. Many women don't get enough folate in their diets, but avocados can go a long way toward fixing that. Half an avocado contains 57 micrograms of folate, 14 percent of the DV.

Moms-to-be aren't the only ones who should be dipping their chips in guacamole, though. Everyone needs folate. It's an essential nutrient for keeping nerves functioning properly. It may also help fight heart disease.

## Getting the Most

**Find fruit from Florida.** Even though the monounsaturated fat in avocados is good for cholesterol, it's not so good for your waistline. To get the nutrients from avocado without all the fat, shop for Florida avocados. They have about two-thirds the calories and half the fat of avocados grown in California. Florida avocados are also much larger than the California variety, weighing it at 1 to 2 pounds each.

**Know when to buy them.** Another way to have avocados with a little less fat is to buy those harvested between November and March. They may have one-third the fat of those picked in September or October.

# Bananas

## A BUNCH OF POTASSIUM

There's something about bananas that makes people laugh. We talk about "going bananas" and "slipping on banana peels." You would think that these yellow-skinned beauties were made for the comedy club.

But here's something that you'll want to take seriously. Studies have shown that the fruit beneath that slippery skin can do wonders for our health. Bananas may help prevent conditions ranging from heart attack and stroke to high blood pressure and infection. They can even help heal ulcers.

Indeed, despite our lack of reverence, we eat bananas by the bunches, with every man, woman, and child tossing down about 27 pounds of them each year. After learning more about bananas' remarkable health benefits, you may want to make that 28.

### BANANAS FOR THE HEART

If the needle on the blood pressure cuff has been inching up in recent years, it may be time for a tropical vacation. If the sun and surf don't bring your pressure down, the bananas sure will.

Bananas are one of nature's best sources of potassium, with each fruit providing about 396 milligrams, 11 percent of the Daily Value (DV) of this essential mineral. Study after study shows that people who eat foods rich in potassium have a significantly lower risk of high blood pressure and related diseases like heart attack and stroke.

Even if you already have high blood pressure, eating plenty of bananas may significantly reduce or even eliminate your need for blood pressure medication, according to scientists at the University of Naples in Italy. Researchers believe that one of the ways that bananas keep blood pressure down is by helping to prevent plaque from sticking to artery walls. They do this by keeping the "bad" low-density lipoprotein cholesterol from oxidizing, a chemical process that makes it more likely to accumulate. That's why bananas may be a good defense against atherosclerosis, or hardening of the arteries, another contributor to high blood pressure, heart attack, and stroke.

And the best part is that you don't have to eat a boatload of bananas to get these benefits, says David B. Young, Ph.D., professor of physiology and biophysics at the University of Mississippi Medical Center in Jackson. Just three to six servings can do the trick.

What's more, researchers from the University of California, San Diego, and the University of Cambridge School of Medicine in England have found that even a single serving of potassium-rich foods such as bananas can lower your risk of stroke by 40 percent.

"Studies show that you can get a significant impact from relatively small changes," says Dr. Young. "My advice would be to think of potassium-rich foods like love and money: You can never get too much."

## STOMACH RELIEF

Though more research needs to be done, bananas may replace antacids in your medicine cabinet as an effective way to quell the inner flames of heartburn and indigestion. Although experts don't know why they work, bananas seem to act as a natural antacid.

In addition, bananas may be helpful both for preventing and treating ulcers. "There have been a few studies showing that bananas may have a protective effect in ulcer treatment," says William Ruderman, M.D., a gastroenterologist in private practice in Orlando, Florida. "But we need more research before we can know for sure."

Scientists suspect that bananas may guard against stomach damage in two ways. First, a chemical in bananas called protease inhibitor appears to be able to kill off harmful, ulcer-causing bacteria before they do their dirty work. Second, bananas seem to stimulate the production of protective mucus, the layer that helps prevent harsh acids from coming into contact with the tender stomach lining.

## RESTORING BALANCE

When you've been run ragged by a case of the runs, it's important that you replenish all the vital fluids and nutrients that diarrhea depletes. And a banana is just the food to do it, says Dr. Ruderman.

"Bananas are a very good source of electrolytes, like potassium, which you lose when you become dehydrated," he explains. Electrolytes are minerals that turn into electrically charged particles in the body, helping to control almost everything that happens inside, from muscle contractions and fluid balance to the beating of the heart.

In addition, bananas contain some pectin, a soluble fiber that acts like a sponge in the digestive tract, absorbing fluids and helping to keep diarrhea in check.

## POWERFUL PREVENTION

Bananas do more than play a role in helping to treat disease. They're also packed with nutrients that can boost immunity, possibly preventing problems before they occur.

One banana delivers 0.6 milligram, 30 percent of the DV for vitamin $B_6$, an essential vitamin that keeps the nervous system working in top condition, makes blood work better, and increases immunity.

A banana also contains 9 milligrams, or 15 percent of the DV of infection-fighting vitamin C, along with 19 micrograms, or 5 percent of the DV of folate, a nutrient that's essential for normal tissue growth and may protect against cancer, heart disease, and birth defects.

# Getting the Most

**Broaden your horizons.** Even if you're not all that fond of bananas as a snack, there are many other ways to get their healing goodness. In Caribbean countries and Central and South America, for example, people frequently add bananas to everyday recipes—everything from meat loaf to casseroles. Because of their mild, slightly sweet taste, bananas work well in almost any recipe.

**Buy a bunch.** One reason that people don't eat a lot of bananas is that they tend to get soft and mushy before you get around to eating them. Here's a trick for keeping them fresh. When bananas are getting soft too quickly, put them in the refrigerator. This will quickly stop the ripening process. (Don't be alarmed when the cold turns the skin black—the fruit inside will still be fresh and tasty.)

On the other hand, when you're waiting for that bunch of green bananas to ripen, it's easy to speed up the process. Put them in a brown paper bag at room temperature. The ethylene gas that bananas produce naturally will speed up the ripening.

# Beans

## SMALL BUT MIGHTY

A generation ago, beans were culinary outcasts. Dusty sacks of pinto and navy beans as well as chickpeas languished on supermarket shelves. Crocks of kidney beans, usually untouched, sat next to cling peaches at steakhouse salad bars. And the three-bean salad at the annual family picnic drew more flies than raves.

Not anymore. Our consumption of beans rose from 5.5 pounds per person in 1974 to 7.3 pounds in 1994. There's a good reason for this surge in popularity. Beans, whether pink, black, red, or speckled, are the ultimate power food—low in fat and high in protein, fiber, and a variety of vitamins and minerals. What's more, studies have found that beans contain a number of powerful compounds that can help lower cholesterol, keep blood sugar under control, and perhaps reduce the risk of certain cancers, including breast cancer.

"Beans are actually little chemical factories with lots of biologically active substances in them, and there's good evidence that eating them may protect against cancer," says Leonard A. Cohen, Ph.D., head of the experimental breast cancer program at the American Health Foundation in Valhalla, New York.

## SENDING CHOLESTEROL SOUTH

While beans aren't the only food that can help lower cholesterol, they're certainly one of the best. Beans are packed with soluble fiber, the same gummy stuff found in apples, barley, and oat bran. When you put soluble fiber in the digestive tract, it helps trap cholesterol-containing bile, removing it from the body before it's absorbed.

"Eating a cup of cooked beans a day can lower total cholesterol about 10 percent in six weeks," says Patti Bazel Geil, R.D., diabetes nutrition educator at the University of Kentucky in Lexington and author of *Magic Beans*. While 10 percent may not seem like much, keep in mind that every 1 percent reduction in total cholesterol means a 2 percent decrease in your risk for heart disease.

Beans can lower cholesterol in just about anyone, but the higher your cholesterol, the better they work. In a study at the University of Kentucky, 20 men with high cholesterol (over 260 milligrams per deciliter of blood) were given about ³/₄ cup of pinto and navy beans a day. The men's total cholesterol dropped an average of 19 percent in three weeks, possibly reducing their heart attack risk by almost 40 percent. Better yet, the dangerous low-density lipoprotein cholesterol—that's the artery-plugging stuff—plunged by 24 percent.

It appears that all beans can help lower cholesterol, even canned baked beans. In another University of Kentucky study, 24 men with high cholesterol ate 1 cup of beans in tomato sauce every day for three weeks. Their total cholesterol dropped 10.4 percent, and their triglycerides (another blood fat that contributes to heart disease) fell 10.8 percent.

Beans play another, less direct role in keeping cholesterol levels down. They're extremely filling, so when you eat beans, you'll have less appetite for other, fattier foods. And eating less fat is critical for keeping cholesterol levels low.

"Beans are a high-fiber food, and high-fiber foods make you feel fuller," says Geil. In fact, one small study found that people who ate a bean puree felt more satisfied for a longer time than those who ate a similar puree made from potatoes.

## KEEPING BLOOD SUGAR STEADY

As anyone with diabetes knows, keeping blood sugar levels steady is the key to keeping this condition under control. "Many people don't realize how good beans are for people with diabetes," says Geil. In fact, eating between ¹/₂ and ³/₄ cup of beans a day has been shown to significantly improve blood sugar control.

Beans are rich in complex carbohydrates. Unlike sugary foods, which dump sugar (glucose) into the bloodstream all at once, complex carbohydrates are digested more slowly. This means that glucose enters your bloodstream a little at a time, helping to keep blood sugar levels steady, says Geil.

In addition, beans are high in soluble fiber. Studies have shown that a diet high in soluble fiber causes the body to produce more insulin receptor sites—tiny "docks" that insulin molecules latch on to. The result is that more insulin gets into individual cells where it's needed, and less is present in the bloodstream, where it can cause problems.

In an English study, people were given either about $1^3/4$ ounces of a variety of beans—including butter beans, kidney beans, black-eyed peas, chickpeas, and lentils—or other high-carbohydrate foods, like bread, pasta, cereals, and grains. After 30 minutes, blood sugar levels in the bean-eaters were almost half that of those who ate other high-carbohydrate foods.

Beans provide another benefit, says Geil. "People with diabetes are four to six times more likely to develop heart disease," she says. "Eating more beans and other foods rich in soluble fiber will help keep their cholesterol low, thereby reducing their risk."

## CANCER-LICKING LEGUMES

Studies suggest that low-fat, fiber-rich beans are some of the best cancer-fighting foods. Beans contain a variety of compounds—lignans, isoflavones, saponins, phytic acid, and protease inhibitors—which, in laboratory studies, have been shown to inhibit cancer cell growth. These compounds appear to keep normal cells from turning cancerous and, in some cases, prevent cancer cells from growing, says Dr. Cohen.

These compounds are as protective to a plant as they are to a human, says Dr. Cohen. "Basically, they're natural insect repellents—they're ways in which plants protect themselves from insects and other predators," he explains. "If beans can block the growth and invasion of insects, molds, and bacteria, it's not surprising that they might also be able to do the same with a cancer cell."

Soybeans (unlike other legumes) are also rich in genistein and daidzen, two compounds that some experts speculate may play a role in preventing cancer. Known as phytoestrogens, these are weaker versions of the estrogen that we produce naturally. Experts believe that these compounds may help reduce the risk of breast and prostate cancer by blocking the activity of testosterone and estrogen, male and female sex hormones that, over time, can spur the growth of cancerous tumors.

Experts have long known that Hispanic women have about half the risk of getting breast cancer that White women face. Studies suggest that beans, which are eaten almost every day in many Hispanic households, may be responsible, says Dr. Cohen.

In one study, Dr. Cohen and his eagues looked at the diets of 214 White, African-American, and Hispanic women. They found that the Hispanic women ate significantly more beans—7.4 servings per week, compared to 4.6 servings per week for the African-American women and less than 3 servings a week for the White women.

"Beans were a major source of fiber for the Hispanic women," says Dr. Cohen. In fact, the Hispanic women consumed nearly 25 percent of their dietary fiber from beans—twice the national average, noted the researchers.

## THE HEALTHY MAN'S MEAT

Beans used to be called the poor man's meat. But a more accurate name would be the healthy man's meat. Like red meat, beans are loaded with protein. Unlike meat, they're light in fat, particularly dangerous, artery-clogging saturated fat.

For example, a cup of black beans contains less than 1 gram of fat. Less than 1 percent of that comes from saturated fat. Three ounces of lean, broiled ground beef, on the other hand, has 15 grams of fat, 22 percent of which is the saturated kind.

Beans are also a great source of essential vitamins and minerals. A half-cup of black beans contains 128 micrograms, or 32 percent of the Daily Value (DV) for folate, a B vitamin that may lower risk of heart disease and fight birth defects. That same cup has 2 milligrams of iron, 11 percent of the DV, and 305 milligrams of potassium, or 9 percent of the DV. Potassium is a mineral that has been shown to help control blood pressure naturally.

## Getting the Most

**Go for the fiber.** While virtually all dried beans are good sources of fiber, some varieties stand out from the pack. Black beans, for example, contain 6 grams of fiber in a half-cup serving. Chickpeas, kidney beans, and lima beans all weigh in at about 7 grams of fiber and black-eyed peas are among the best, with about 8 grams of fiber.

**Enjoy them canned.** Don't have time to soak and cook dried beans? No problem. Canned beans are just as good for you as the dried kind, says Geil. They're higher in sodium, however, so drain and rinse canned beans well before using them.

**Use gas-deflating spices.** Has the fear of uncomfortable and embarrassing gas kept you from reaping beans' nutritional benefits? Try spicing them with a pinch of summer savory or a teaspoon of ground ginger. According to some university studies, these spices may help reduce beans' gas-producing effects.

# Beets

## BETTER LIVING THROUGH BORSCHT

When you think of healthy cuisine, foods from the Great Bear—Russia—don't come immediately to mind.

It's little wonder, really. We don't usually think of such things as butter-laden cabbage and potatoes, washed down with a slug of vodka, as haute cuisine—or healthy cuisine.

Yet there's one traditional Russian dish that deserves a second look: borscht. Served hot or cold, this sweet crimson soup is made from fresh beets, and that means that it's brimming with nutrients that can fight birth defects, make blood work better and perhaps even stave off cancer.

### GIVING CANCER THE RED FLAG

Folk medicine is full of stories about using beets and beet juice for fighting cancer. Though much more research needs to be done, some scientists suspect that the compound that gives beets their rich, crimson color—betacyanin—is also a powerful tumor-fighting agent.

"Beet juice is used in Europe for the treatment of cancer," says Eleonore Blaurock-Busch, Ph.D., president of Trace Minerals International in Boulder, Colorado. "The pigment found in beets may have anti-cancer properties."

In one of the few studies on beets' effectiveness against cancer, researchers tested beet juice, along with the juices of other vegetables and fruits, against common cancer-causing chemicals. Compared to other juices used in the study, beet juice ranked close to the top in preventing cell mutations that commonly lead to cancer.

"When it comes to fighting cancer, beets aren't as well-studied as other vegetables, like broccoli," notes Dr. Blaurock-Busch. "But there's certainly enough evidence to warrant including them in your diet. Plus, they're nutritious. And they taste good."

## A FONT OF FOLATE

If there's one nutrient that women often don't get enough of, it's the B vitamin folate. They just don't eat enough lentils, spinach, or other folate-rich foods to get the 400 micrograms they need each day.

Meeting the daily requirement for folate is essential for normal tissue growth and perhaps for protecting against heart disease and certain cancers. Plus, doctors have found that folate is a pregnant woman's best friend because it helps protect against birth defects.

A half-cup of boiled, sliced beets contains 45 micrograms of folate, nearly 11 percent of the Daily Value (DV).

## INCREASING IRON STORES

For providing iron, beets can't match such mineral powerhouses as lean beef. But if you're among the millions of Americans who are cutting back on meat or giving it up entirely, then boning up on beets is one way to go.

"Many vegetarians get some of their iron from beets," says Dr. Blaurock-Busch. Each cup of boiled, sliced beets delivers 1 milligram of iron, about 6 percent of the Recommended Dietary Allowance (RDA) for women and 10 percent of the RDA for men.

Even though beets don't contain a huge amount of iron, they do contain vitamin C—9 milligrams in a 1-cup serving, 15 percent of the DV. This helps in two ways: First, it helps the body absorb more iron than it normally would. Second, vitamin C is helpful in its own right. As an antioxidant vitamin, it sweeps up free radicals, cell-damaging oxygen molecules that have been linked to certain cancers, heart disease, and a variety of other conditions.

# Getting the Most

**Cook them lightly.** Studies show that the anti-tumor power of beets is diminished by heat. So you'll want to cook them lightly to get the most effectiveness.

**Try the canned kind.** One of the neat things about beets is that they're nearly as nutritious out of a can as they are fresh from the ground. So you can enjoy their health benefits in and out of season.

# Broccoli

## KING OF THE CRUCIFERS

$A$sk researchers to name the one vegetable that they buy specifically for cancer prevention, and they'll say that broccoli is the one.

It's difficult to overestimate broccoli's healing powers. This crisp, delicious member of the cruciferous family has been shown to fend off a host of serious conditions, including heart disease and cancer.

### DOUBLE CANCER PROTECTION

Broccoli's impressive power as a cancer fighter is due in part to its two-pronged attack. It contains not just one but two separate compounds—indole-3-carbinol (or I3C, for short) and sulforaphane—that help sweep up cancer-causing substances before they have a chance to do harm.

The compound I3C, which is also found in cabbage and brussels sprouts, is particularly effective against breast cancer. In laboratory studies, I3C has been found to lower levels of harmful estrogens that can promote tumor growth in hormone-sensitive cells, like breast cells.

While I3C is working against hormone-induced cancers, sulforaphane is offering protection on another front, by boosting the production of cancer-blocking enzymes, says Thomas Kensler, Ph.D., professor in the department of environmental health sciences in the School of Public Health at Johns Hopkins University in Baltimore.

In one pioneering study, Dr. Kensler and his colleagues at Johns Hopkins University exposed 145 laboratory animals to a powerful cancer-causing agent. Twenty-five of the animals had not received any special treatment, while the rest were fed high doses of sulforaphane. After 50 days, 68 percent of the unprotected animals had breast tumors, compared with only 26 percent of those given the sulforaphane.

It is no wonder that researchers put broccoli at the top of their lists of nutritional superstars. "We know that people who eat lots of cruciferous vegetables, like broccoli, are protected from every kind of cancer," says Jon Michnovicz, M.D., Ph.D., president of the Foundation for Preventive Oncology and the Institute for Hormone Research, both in New York City. Broccoli and other crucifers are particularly helpful when it comes to preventing cancers of the colon, breast, and prostate gland, he adds.

## A BOOST FROM BETA-CAROTENE

While much recent research has focused on "exotic" compounds like sulforaphane, broccoli is also chock-full of more common, but still powerful, compounds like beta-carotene. This nutrient, which the body converts to vitamin A, is one of the antioxidants. That is, it helps prevent disease by sweeping up harmful, cell-damaging oxygen molecules that naturally accumulate in the body. High levels of beta-carotene have been linked to lower rates of heart attack, certain cancers, and cataracts.

Broccoli is an excellent source of beta-carotene, providing about 0.7 milligram in a half-cup cooked serving. This provides 7 to 12 percent of the recommended daily amount.

## SUPPORTING PLAYERS

Broccoli isn't called the king of the crucifers for nothing. Along with beta-carotene, sulforaphane, I3C, and broccoli contains a variety of other nutrients, each of which can help fend off a host of conditions, from heart disease to osteoporosis.

For example, just a half-cup of chopped, cooked broccoli contains almost 100 percent of the Daily Value for vitamin C. This vitamin has been proven in studies to help boost immunity and fight diseases like heart disease and cancer.

Broccoli also ranks up there with diamonds as a woman's best friend. It's one of the best vegetable sources of calcium, packing in 72 milligrams per cooked cup—about a quarter of the amount in an 8-ounce glass of skim milk. Calcium is well-documented as the single most important nutrient that women need to keep osteoporosis (the breaking down of bones) at bay.

Broccoli is also rich in folate, a nutrient that's essential for normal tissue growth and that studies show may protect against cancer, heart disease, and birth defects. Women, especially those who take birth control pills, are often low in this vital nutrient.

Finally, if you're looking to keep your digestive system running smoothly, make broccoli your fuel of choice, experts advise. A half-cup provides 2 grams of fiber, which is a proven protector against constipation, hemorrhoids, colon cancer, diabetes, high cholesterol, heart disease, and obesity.

Experts aren't yet sure how much broccoli you need to maximize its healing potential. Dr. Kensler advises eating at least five servings of fruits and vegetables a day, while reaching for this crunchy crucifer whenever you can.

## Getting the Most

**Heat it—but just a little.** While gently cooking broccoli helps release some of its protective compounds, overheating it can destroy others. "Carotenoids like beta-carotene are preserved by heat, but the indoles, like I3C, don't withstand a lot of heat," explains Dr. Michnovicz. "Light steaming is a great way to cook broccoli. And microwaving is okay, too."

**Buy it purple.** You'll notice at the supermarket that broccoli is sometimes so dark that it's almost purple. That's good. The dark color means that it has more beta-carotene, experts say. If it's yellowish, on the other hand, skip it. That means that it's old, and its nutritional clock is running down.

**Keep it cool.** When buying fresh broccoli, the nutritional value will be higher if you buy it chilled and keep it cold. Properly stored, it will keep for up to four days. Frozen broccoli, of course, will keep longer; and it provides virtually the same amount of nutrients as fresh.

# Brussels Sprouts

## GOOD THINGS IN SMALL PACKAGES

If any one food has the reputation for being "the thing on your plate you'd most like to slip to your dog," it might be brussels sprouts. Just say the name and people start crinkling their noses.

Well, believe it or not, brussels sprouts have gotten a lot tastier during the past decade. What's more, scientists have found that they're even better for you than they ever imagined.

## NEW TASTE IN THE MARKETPLACE

Brussels sprouts are miniature members of the cabbage family. And while the brussels sprouts of yore were often strong and bitter, the taste has literally changed, says Steve Bontadelli, a brussels sprouts grower in Santa Cruz, California.

The taste problem originally began when brussels sprouts growers started using machines instead of harvesting sprouts by hand. To make machine harvesting easier, they developed a new strain of sprouts. Unfortunately, these "new and improved" plants yielded some really bitter sprouts, recalls Bontadelli.

"It wasn't until the past 10 years or so that brussels sprouts growers started changing the hybrids to make them taste better," he says. "Today they are much sweeter and milder."

So now you'll be smacking your lips instead of holding your nose when you spoon these health-saving leafy nuggets onto your plate. Taste aside, brussels sprouts are packed with plant chemicals that provide protection against major league diseases like cancer and heart disease.

## Belgium's Burly Cancer-Beaters

Like other cruciferous vegetables, brussels sprouts are chock-full of natural plant compounds called phytonutrients, which may help protect against cancer. These compounds may be particularly effective against common cancers like those of the breast and colon.

One of the key protective compounds in brussels sprouts is sulforaphane. Sulforaphane triggers the release of enzymes that help rid your body's cells of toxic wastes and reduce your risk for cancer, says Jon Michnovicz, M.D., Ph.D., president of the Foundation for Preventive Oncology and the Institute for Hormone Research, both in New York City.

In a groundbreaking study at Johns Hopkins University in Baltimore, scientists exposed 145 laboratory animals to a powerful cancer-causing agent called DMBA. Twenty-five of the animals had not received any special treatment, while the rest had been fed high doses of sulforaphane. Fifty days later, 68 percent of the unprotected animals had breast tumors, compared with only 26 percent of those that received the sulforaphane.

Brussels sprouts contain another protective phytonutrient called indole-3-carbinol, or I3C. This compound works as an anti-estrogen, meaning it helps sweep up your body's harmful estrogens before they contribute to the growth of cancer cells. It also helps boost the production of certain enzymes that help clear cancer-causing toxins from the body. "Indoles are probably very useful against colon, breast, and prostate cancers," explains Dr. Michnovicz. "And population studies show that they probably protect against other cancers as well."

In one small study, researchers in the Netherlands found that people who ate more than 10 ounces of brussels sprouts (about 14 sprouts) a day for one week had levels of protective cancer-fighting enzymes in their colon that were, on average, 23 percent higher than people who did not eat brussels sprouts.

In another study, five people ate more than 10 ounces of brussels sprouts a day for three weeks, while another five avoided the sprouts and other similar vegetables. At the end of the study, the sprout-eating group had 28 percent less wear and tear to their DNA. It's a promising find, say experts, because the healthier you keep your DNA, the healthier you stay.

## BRUSSELS FOR YOUR BOWELS

Aside from all the "science-y" compounds in brussels sprouts, there are also plenty of good old-fashioned vitamins, minerals, and other substances that can help fight off cancer, heart disease, high cholesterol, and a host of other problems.

Topping this list is fiber. Brussels sprouts are a good source of fiber, with about 3 grams in a half-cup serving. You'd have to eat more than two slices of whole-grain bread to get the amount of fiber in a half-cup of these little green gems.

Eating your daily fill of brussels sprouts can help you avoid all the conditions that a diet rich in fiber is known to prevent, like constipation, hemorrhoids, and other digestive complaints.

A half-cup of brussels sprouts provides 48 milligrams of immunity-building vitamin C, more than 80 percent of the Daily Value (DV). It also provides 47 micrograms of folate, about 12 percent of the DV. Folete is essential for normal tissue growth, and studies show that it may protect against cancer, heart disease, and birth defects. Women, especially those on birth control pills, often have low levels of this important vitamin.

# Getting the Most

**Steam them.** Though you'll lose some nutrients during the cooking process, raw brussels sprouts just don't go down well. Gently steaming brussels sprouts will help release some of their healing compounds. But don't steam them too long; cooking sprouts until they're mushy makes them lose too much vitamin C, along with other valuable phytonutrients. Plus, overcooking gives them a bitter kick, says Dr. Michnovicz.

# Cabbage Family

## A HEAD ABOVE THE REST

Ancient Roman healers thought that they could cure breast cancer by rubbing on pastes made from cabbage. A few years ago, modern scientists would have dismissed that practice as so much folklore. Now they're not so sure.

"Studies have shown that if you make cabbage into a paste and rub it on the backs of laboratory animals, you can prevent tumors from developing," says Jon Michnovicz, M.D., Ph.D., president of the Foundation for Preventive Oncology and the Institute for Hormone Research, both in New York City.

Of course, the best way to absorb the healing properties of cabbage is simply to eat it. Cabbage not only fights off a variety of cancers but also contains a wealth of nutrients that can ward off heart disease, digestive problems, and other conditions, according to research.

### CABBAGE AGAINST CANCER

Like other members of the cruciferous vegetable family, cabbage contains several compounds that studies show can help prevent cancers from occurring. It's particularly effective in preventing cancers of the breast, prostate gland, and colon.

There are two compounds in particular that scientists believe make cabbage a particularly potent cancer-fighting food. The first of these, indole-3-carbinol, or I3C, is especially effective against breast cancer, research shows. The compound acts as an anti-estrogen, meaning that it sweeps up harmful estrogens that have been linked to breast cancer.

In one study, researchers gave a group of Israeli women about a third of a head of cabbage a day for three months. After five days of eating the cabbage-fortified diet, the women's levels of harmful hormones dropped significantly.

"In my studies, there was no doubt that if we gave women pure I3C, it would work," says Dr. Michnovicz. "But this study showed that for the average person, eating cabbage or a cabbagelike vegetable, like broccoli, would have the same effect."

For even more protection, try replacing your usual cabbage with bok choy, or Chinese cabbage. Laboratory research has found that a compound in bok choy called brassinin may help prevent breast tumors.

Cabbage contains another compound, sulforaphane, which has been shown to block cancer by stepping up the production of tumor-preventing enzymes in the body.

In a pioneering study at Johns Hopkins University in Baltimore, scientists exposed 145 laboratory animals to a powerful cancer-causing chemical. Twenty-five of the animals had not received any special treatment, while the rest had been fed high doses of sulforaphane. Fifty days later, 68 percent of the unprotected animals had breast tumors, compared with only 26 percent of those given high doses of sulforaphane.

Sulforaphane makes cabbage a particularly prized fighter in the battle against colon cancer, adds Dr. Michnovicz, because it stimulates levels of an enzyme called glutathione in the colon, which researchers believe sweeps toxins out of the body before they have a chance to do damage.

Eating any kind of cabbage on a regular basis will probably lower your risk for cancer. Yet a gold-medal winner is savoy cabbage, say researchers. Savoy contains not only I3C and sulforaphane but also four other tongue-twisting phytonutrients—beta-sitosterol, pheophytin-a, nonacosane, and nonacosanone—that studies show are powerful contenders against potential cancer-causing agents.

## ANTIOXIDANT PROTECTION

You've heard a lot about antioxidants such as vitamins C and E and beta-carotene, which help ward off disease by mopping up harmful oxygen molecules called free radicals that naturally accumulate in the body.

Members of the cabbage family are packed with these nutritious compounds. Particularly good are cabbages like bok choy and savoy, which are super sources of beta-carotene, a nutrient that other cabbages don't have in abundance. High blood levels of beta-carotene are related to lower incidences of heart attacks, certain types of cancers, and cataracts.

Not only are these cabbages high in beta-carotene; they're also a good source of vitamin C, which has been shown to boost immunity as well as reduce blood pressure and fight heart disease. A half-cup serving of raw bok choy provides 16 milligrams of vitamin C, 27 percent of the Daily Value (DV), while the same amount of raw savoy cabbage supplies 11 milligrams, 18 percent of the DV.

Both bok choy and savoy cabbage are also decent sources of folate, with a half-cup of either providing about 35 micrograms, or 9 percent of the DV. Your body uses folate for normal tissue growth. Studies show that folate also may protect against cancer, heart disease, and birth defects. Research shows that women are at high risk for folate deficiency, especially if they take birth control pills.

# Getting the Most

**Keep a cool head.** Boiling cabbage removes about half the valuable indoles, experts say. To preserve these compounds at maximum levels, experts advise eating cabbage raw—mixed in with a green salad, for example, or concentrated in coleslaw.

**Enjoy the variety.** To get the healing benefits of cabbage several times a week without getting bored, explore the different varieties. Green, red, and savoy cabbages, along with bok choy, all are high in protective compounds. They can be eaten raw in coleslaw, slow-cooked in soup, or wrapped around your favorite filling.

**Stock up.** We often avoid stocking up on fresh produce because it can go bad so quickly. Never fear with cabbage. A head of cabbage will keep for up to 10 days in the crisper drawer, making it easy to eat a little bit each day without worrying about it spoiling.

# Carrots

## GOOD FOR THE EYES—AND MORE

As kids, we all heard how good carrots are for our eyes. But nowadays, researchers are seeing carrots in a whole new light.

The healing potential of carrots goes far beyond their ability to help our vision. They contain a variety of compounds that may help prevent certain cancers, lower cholesterol, and prevent heart attacks.

### CAROTENE'S NAMESAKE

The same substance that gives carrots their brash orange color is also responsible for providing many of their health benefits. Carrots are rich in beta-carotene, an antioxidant compound that fights free radicals, the unstable molecules in the body that contribute to conditions ranging from heart disease and cancer to macular degeneration, the leading cause of vision loss in older adults.

Research suggests that the more antioxidants we get in our diets, the less likely we are to die of cancer. In a study of 1,556 middle-age men, researchers from the University of Texas School of Public Health in Houston and Rush–Presbyterian–St. Luke's Medical Center and Northwestern University Medical School, both in Chicago, found that those with the highest levels of beta-carotene and vitamin C in their diets had a 37 percent lower risk of death from cancer than the men with the lowest levels.

Even when vitamin C isn't added to the mix, beta-carotene has powerful effects. Large population studies have shown that having low levels of beta-carotene leaves people more open to developing certain cancers, especially those of the lungs and stomach. In addition, evidence shows that eating large amounts of carrots and other fruits and vegetables rich in beta-carotene and related compounds may reduce the risk of heart disease.

"A half-cup serving of cooked carrots contains 12 milligrams of beta-carotene, about twice the amount you need to get the benefits," says Paul Lachance, Ph.D., professor of nutrition and chairman of the department of food science at Rutgers University in New Brunswick, New Jersey.

It's not only beta-carotene that gives carrots their protective edge. They contain another antioxidant, alpha-carotene, that also appears to help fight cancer. In one study, researchers at the National Cancer Institute in Bethesda, Maryland, found that lung cancer occurred more often in men with low intakes of alpha-carotene than in men who got more.

## BETTER VISION

The beta-carotene in carrots does double duty. It converts to vitamin A in the body and helps improve vision. This eye appeal is so well-known that British researchers in World War II cultivated carrots that were especially high in beta-carotene to help pilots see better at night.

Vitamin A helps vision by forming a purple pigment that the eye needs in order to be able to see in dim light. This pigment, called rhodopsin, is located in the light-sensitive area of the retina. The more vitamin A you get, the more rhodopsin your body is able to produce. Conversely, people with low levels of vitamin A may have night blindness, which can make it difficult to drive after dark or to find a seat in a dark theater. True vitamin A deficiencies, however, are rare in this country.

# Getting the Most

**Add a little fat.** Beta-carotene needs a small amount of fat to make the trip through the intestinal wall and into your body, says John Erdman, Ph.D., director of the division of nutritional sciences at the University of Illinois in Urbana. So the next time you're serving carrot sticks, you may want to accompany them with a small amount of a dip such as ranch dressing.

**Eat them cooked.** While many foods are more nutritious raw than cooked, carrots benefit from a little cooking. The reason is that carrots have a lot of dietary fiber—over 2 grams in one carrot—which traps the beta-carotene, says Dr. Erdman. "There's quite a bit of beta-carotene there, but it is very difficult to get it out," he says. Cooking carrots helps free beta-carotene from the fiber cells, making it easier for your body to absorb.

**Save the nutrients.** One problem with cooking carrots is that some of the nutrients escape into the cooking water, says Carol Boushey, R.D., Ph.D., assistant professor of food and nutrition at Southern Illinois University in Carbondale. To get nutrients into your body instead of pouring them down the sink, try reusing the cooking water—in a sauce, for example, or for moistening mashed potatoes.

**Enjoy some juice.** Another way to release more of the beta-carotene from carrots is to make a carrot cocktail. Processing carrots in a blender breaks apart the fibers, allowing the beta-carotene to get out, says Dr. Erdman.

**Try some babies.** Not everyone enjoys the tough texture and somewhat bitter taste of grown carrots. An alternative is to have baby carrots, Dr. Boushey says. "They are easier to eat because they don't have a tough core."

**Trim them well.** When you buy carrots with the greenery still on them, it's important to trim it off before storing them. Otherwise, those pretty, leafy tops will act like nutrient vampires, sucking out the vitamins and moisture before you eat the carrots.

# Cauliflower

## A WHITE KNIGHT AGAINST CANCER

$M$ark Twain once called cauliflower "a cabbage with a college education"—a bit more refined, perhaps, but essentially the same plain-Jane vegetable. What Twain didn't know is just how valuable cauliflower is in our quest for good health. (If he had, Huckleberry Finn and Jim might have spent their days eating raw cauliflower instead of greasy catfish fillets.) Like other members of the cruciferous family, cauliflower is loaded with nutrients that seem to wage war against a host of diseases, including cancer.

### FORMIDABLE FLORETS

Although cauliflower's darker-hued brother, broccoli, generally hogs the healing spotlight, cauliflower has its share of cancer-preventing powers, says Jon Michnovicz, M.D., Ph.D., president of the Foundation for Preventive Oncology and the Institute for Hormone Research, both in New York City.

Researchers have found two potent munitions in cauliflower's cancer-fighting arsenal: the phytonutrients sulforaphane and indole-3-carbinol, or I3C. These compounds, which are found in all cruciferous vegetables, may be the reason that studies consistently show that folks who make a habit of crunching crucifers are less likely to get cancer.

In one study, scientists at Johns Hopkins University in Baltimore exposed 145 laboratory animals to high doses of a cancer-causing agent. Of those, 120 were given high levels of protective sulforaphane. Fifty days later, 68 percent of the unprotected animals had breast tumors, compared with only 26 percent of those that received the sulforaphane.

Sulforaphane works by stepping up the production of enzymes in your body that sweep toxins out the door before they can damage your body's cells, making them cancerous, explains Dr. Michnovicz.

Cauliflower's other tumor-squelching compound, I3C, works as an anti-estrogen, explains Dr. Michnovicz. In other words, it reduces levels of harmful estrogens that can foster tumor growth in hormone-sensitive cells, like those in the breasts and prostate gland.

"That's why, although studies show that people who eat cruciferous vegetables are protected from all kinds of cancers, these foods are probably most useful for fighting cancers of the colon, breast, and prostate," says Dr. Michnovicz.

## IMMUNE POWER

Cauliflower does more than protect against cancer. It's also packed with vitamin C and folate, two nutrients that are well-known for keeping your immune system in peak condition.

Just three uncooked florets of this crisp crucifer supply 67 percent of the Daily Value (DV) for vitamin C—more than the amount in a tangerine or a white grapefruit. By upping your level of vitamin C, along with other antioxidant vitamins like vitamin E and beta-carotene, you can keep your immune system strong while staving off a host of conditions, among them heart disease, cancer, and cataracts.

Cauliflower also contains folate, which is important because too little folate is perhaps the country's most common nutritional deficiency. Three uncooked florets of cauliflower provide 9 percent of the DV for folate.

Since folate can help blood work more efficiently, it's often recommended for preventing anemia. In addition, research has shown that folate is essential for normal tissue growth. Not getting enough folate over the long term could set the stage for diseases like cancer and heart disease down the road, say researchers.

## Getting the Most

**Look for a clear complexion.** Don't buy cauliflower if it has brown spots on its ivory (or purple) florets. That means that it's already past its nutritional peak.

**Enjoy it raw.** To keep cauliflower's cancer-fighting indoles intact, keep it out of the heat, advises Dr. Michnovicz. Your best bet is either eating it raw or cooking it quickly in a steamer, wok, or microwave, he says. Boiling is the worst way to cook this crucifer since you lose about half of the valuable indoles in the process, he says.

# Celery

## STALKS OF PROTECTION

The ancient Romans, notorious party animals that they were, wore wreaths of celery to protect them from hangovers, which may explain the practice of putting celery sticks in Bloody Marys.

While there's no evidence that donning a celery chapeau will save you from the consequences of having one too many, celery does have other healing properties. This member of the parsley family contains compounds that may help lower blood pressure and perhaps help prevent cancer. Celery is also a good source of insoluble fiber as well as a number of essential nutrients, including potassium, vitamin C, and calcium.

## CHOMP DOWN ON BLOOD PRESSURE

Celery has been used for centuries in Asia as a folk remedy for high blood pressure. In the United States, it took one man with high blood pressure and persistence to persuade researchers at the University of Chicago Medical Center to put this remedy to the scientific test.

The story began when a man named Mr. Le was diagnosed with mild high blood pressure. Rather than cutting back on salt as his doctor advised, he began eating a quarter-pound (about four stalks) of celery per day. Within a week his blood pressure had dropped from 158/96 to 118/82.

William J. Elliott, M.D., Ph.D., who was then assistant professor of medicine and pharmacological and physiological science at the University of Chicago, decided to put celery to the test. Researchers injected test animals with a small amount of 3-n-butyl phthalide, a chemical compound found in celery. Within a week, the animals' blood pressures dropped an average of 12 to 14 percent.

"Phthalide was found to relax the muscles of the arteries that regulate blood pressure, allowing the vessels to dilate," says Dr. Elliott. The chemical also reduced blood levels of "stress hormones," called cate-cholamines. This may be helpful because stress hormones typically raise blood pressure by causing blood vessels to constrict.

If you have high blood pressure and would like to give celery a try, try this strategy recommended by Asian folk practitioners. Eat four to five stalks every day for a week, then stop for three weeks. Then start over and eat celery for another week.

But don't overdo it and start eating celery by the pound, Dr. Elliott warns. Celery does contain sodium—about 35 milligrams per stalk—and for some people this can cause blood pressure to go up rather than down.

## BLOCKING CANCER CELLS

Who'd have thought that crunching celery might help prevent cancer? Celery contains a number of compounds that researchers believe may help prevent cancer cells from spreading.

For starters, celery contains compounds called acetylenics. "Acetylenics have been shown to stop the growth of tumor cells," says Robert Rosen, Ph.D., associate director of the Center for Advanced Food Technology at Cook College, Rutgers University, in New Brunswick, New Jersey.

In addition, celery also contains compounds called phenolic acids, which block the action of hormonelike substances called prostaglandins. Some prostaglandins are thought to encourage the growth of tumor cells, says Dr. Rosen.

## Getting the Most

**Leave on the leaves.** While celery stalks are certainly a healthful snack, it's the leaves that contain the most nutrients.

**Eat it the way you like it.** While many foods lose nutrients when they are cooked, most of the compounds in celery hold up well during cooking. Eating a cup of celery, raw or cooked, provides about 9 milligrams of vitamin C, 15 percent of the Daily Value (DV); 426 milligrams of potassium, 12 percent of the DV; and 60 milligrams of calcium, 6 percent of the DV.

**Sprinkle on the seeds.** Celery seeds, which are found in the spice section of supermarkets, provide a nutritional bonus. One tablespoon of seeds, which can be added to soups, stews, or casseroles, contains 3 milligrams of iron, 17 percent of the DV.

# Chili Peppers

## RED-HOT HEALERS

According to an old saying, "Whatever doesn't kill you makes you stronger." This might be the perfect motto for the chili pepper. Not only can many people withstand the heat, they actually enjoy it. Maybe it's the fun of wowing people who can't stomach any condiment stronger than ketchup. Maybe it's the rush they experience when they bite into these pungent pods. But whatever the reason, chili pepper fans savor the heat at every opportunity, not just in traditional favorites like tacos and burritos but also in foods such as omelets, stews, and even salads.

More is involved than just a little culinary spice. These thermogenic morsels are prized around the globe for their healing power as well as their firepower. Hot chilies have long been used as natural remedies for coughs, colds, sinusitis, and bronchitis, says Irwin Ziment, M.D., professor of medicine at the University of California, Los Angeles. There's some evidence that they can help lower low-density lipoprotein (LDL) cholesterol, the type associated with stroke, high blood pressure, and heart disease. There's also some evidence that chilies can help prevent—of all things—stomach ulcers.

## HEAT UP A COLD

Chili-lovers have long asserted that hot peppers, from serranos to jalapeños, are the ultimate decongestant, clearing a stuffy nose in the time it takes to gasp "Yow!" In fact, the fiery bite of hot chilies (or chili-based condiments like Tabasco sauce) can work as well as over-the-counter cold remedies, says Dr. Ziment. "Some of the foods used to fight respiratory diseases for centuries, including hot peppers, are very similar to the drugs we now use."

The stuff that makes hot peppers so nose-clearing good is capsaicin, a plant chemical that gives hot peppers their sting. Chemically, capsaicin is similar to a drug called guaifenesin, which is used in many over-the-counter and prescription cold remedies such as Robitussin, says Dr. Ziment.

Of course, eating a chili pepper has more of an immediate impact than taking a spoonful of medicine. When hot pepper meets tongue, the brain is slammed with an onslaught of nerve messages from the mouth, tongue, back of the throat, and stomach. The brain responds to this "Ow!" message by stimulating secretion-producing glands that line the airways. The result is a flood of fluids that makes your eyes water, your nose run, and the mucus in your lungs loosen, says Dr. Ziment.

In other words, chili peppers are a natural decongestant and expectorant. "Helping break up congestion and clearing the sinuses are common traits of any hot foods," explains Dr. Ziment.

It doesn't take a lot of pepper to get the healing benefits. Adding 10 drops of hot-pepper sauce to a bowl of chicken soup can be very effective, says Paul Bosland, Ph.D., professor in the department of horticulture at New Mexico State University in Las Cruces and founder of the Chile Pepper Institute at the university. "Most of us here in New Mexico do this when we're sick," he says. "We all feel better after we've had a little bit of chili pepper."

Dr. Ziment recommends treating a cold with a warm-water gargle to which you've added 10 drops of Tabasco sauce. "This remedy can be quite effective, particularly if you want to clear your sinuses," he says.

## HELP FOR HEART AND STOMACH

Besides unblocking clogged airways, chilies may also cut blood cholesterol, says Earl Mindell, R.Ph., Ph.D., pharmacist and professor of nutrition at Pacific Western University in Los Angeles and author of *Earl Mindell's Food as Medicine*. "When laboratory animals were fed a diet high in capsaicin and low in saturated fat, it helped reduce their 'bad' LDL cholesterol," says Dr. Mindell.

Eating chili peppers also appears to have a blood-thinning effect. Researchers at Max Planck Institute in Germany found that chilies can hinder the formation of blood clots by increasing the amount of time it takes for blood to coagulate. This could play a role in helping prevent blood clots that lead to heart attack and stroke, says Dr. Mindell.

For years, doctors advised people prone to ulcers to abstain from spicy foods. Research now suggests the opposite: that chili peppers may help prevent ulcers from occurring.

Capsaicin appears to shield the stomach lining from ulcer-causing acids and alcohol by stimulating the flow of protective digestive juices. Researchers at National University Hospital in Singapore found that people who consumed the most chili powder had the fewest ulcers, leading them to speculate that chili, or capsaicin, was the protective factor.

## RED-HOT VITAMINS

Getting more hot chilies into your diet may strengthen your personal anti-aging arsenal. That's because they're a rich source of the antioxidants vitamin C and beta-carotene (which is converted into vitamin A in the body).

These antioxidants help protect the body by "neutralizing" free radicals, harmful oxygen molecules that naturally accumulate in the body and cause cell damage. Upping your intake of antioxidant vitamins, researchers believe, may help prevent damage that can lead to cancer, heart disease, and stroke as well as such things as arthritis and a weakened immune system.

One red chili packs 3 milligrams of beta-carotene, between 30 and 50 percent of the amount recommended by most experts. Studies show that people who consume more beta-carotene-rich foods get less cancer and heart disease. One chili also contains almost 5,000 international units of vitamin A, 100 percent of the Daily Value (DV), and more than 100 milligrams of vitamin C, nearly twice the DV.

# Getting the Most

**Enjoy them raw.** Although raw chilies can be uncomfortably hot for some people, that's the best way to get the most vitamin C; cooking destroys the stores of this vitamin, says Dr. Bosland.

On the other hand, capsaicin isn't affected by heating, so if that's what you're after—to help relieve congestion, for example—cook the peppers to your taste.

**Munch the membrane.** Inside the chili is a thin membrane that connects the seeds to the flesh. Most of the capsaicin in chili peppers is located in the membrane, experts say.

**Preserve the powder.** Storing chili powder at room temperature will eventually deplete its beta-carotene. "Keep chili powder in a dark, cool place, like in the freezer," says Dr. Bosland. Buying whole pods and grinding them as needed will also help preserve the beta-carotene, he says.

**Eat for comfort.** The hottest chili pepper isn't necessarily the most healing, so don't make yourself suffer. From wild to mild, here are a few chilies you may want to try.

- Habanero pepper and Scotch bonnet are among the most mouth-blistering peppers.
- Jalapeño and Fresno peppers weigh in at 50 percent firepower, compared to the habanero.
- Hungarian cherry and Anaheim peppers emit more of a glow than a flame and are a good choice for tamer palates.

# Cranberries
## A Sauce for All Seasons

Pity the lowly cranberry. Like swallows returning to San Juan Capistrano, this Thanksgiving staple finds its way back into our diet every year—then gets lost after the holiday season is over.

And that's a pity. Cranberries contain a number of compounds that show early promise against cancer and heart disease. What's more, cranberry juice has finally earned the scientific stamp of approval for its traditional role in relieving bladder infections.

### A Role against Cancer

Along with raspberries, strawberries, and blackberries, cranberries are a good source of ellagic acid, an antioxidant compound that has raised high hopes in cancer researchers.

In laboratory tests, ellagic acid has been shown to help prevent mutations in DNA, the genetic stuff that instructs our cells how to function. In addition, ellagic acid has been shown to disarm cancer-causing agents and also to help prevent tumors from growing.

Indeed, one tantalizing aspect of this compound is its apparent ability to battle carcinogens on both ends—before and after they take hold. "Ellagic acid has what we call anti-initiating activity. It inhibits the genetic damage that starts the cancer process," says Gary D. Stoner, Ph.D., director of the cancer chemoprevention program at the Ohio State University Comprehensive Cancer Center in Columbus. Even after a carcinogen has been introduced into cells, he says, ellagic acid helps prevent the cells from becoming cancerous.

Pure ellagic acid—the form in which it's used in laboratory studies—doesn't get into the bloodstream very well. However, Dr. Stoner's research suggests that this compound is better absorbed in its natural state in food—good news for those who enjoy their cranberries year-round.

61

## POWER FROM FLAVONOIDS

Another way in which cranberries will help keep you healthy is by putting more flavonoids into your diet. Flavonoids are plant pigments that put the reds and yellows into fruits and vegetables and that have powerful antioxidant abilities—that is, they help block damage from free radicals, which are harmful oxygen molecules that can lead to cancer, heart disease, and other serious conditions.

Cranberries contain two powerful flavonoids—quercetin and myricetin. The darker cranberry varieties, like Stevens, Early Black, and Ben Lear, contain a third compound called kaempferol. Each of these compounds has been shown in studies to help prevent genetic changes that can lead to cancer.

Here's a bonus. Flavonoids, in general, and quercetin, in particular, are thought to play a role in preventing artery disease, perhaps because their antioxidant ability helps prevent damage to the linings of blood vessels.

Large studies in Finland, the Netherlands, and the United Kingdom have shown that people with very low intakes of flavonoids have high risks of coronary disease. In one study of middle-age men in the Dutch town of Zutphen, those who ate a lot of fruits and vegetables—and consequently had a high intake of flavonoids—had a 73 percent lower risk of stroke than men who consumed few fruits and vegetables.

## HELP FOR URINARY COMPLAINTS

For ages now, grandmothers and mothers—and a few wise doctors—have recommended cranberry juice to clear up urinary tract infections. Now, scientists are coming on board. A 1994 Harvard Medical School study of elderly women found that those who drank about 10 ounces of cranberry juice cocktail daily for six months had significantly lower amounts of bacteria in their urine and were almost 60 percent less likely to develop infections than women who drank a noncranberry impostor.

What's more, among women who already had infections, those drinking cranberry juice were nearly 75 percent more likely to have the infections clear up.

One long-held belief was that if you could make urine more acidic, bacteria would have a tougher time growing. This was thought to be why cranberry juice helped prevent urinary tract infections. Following the same line of reasoning, doctors sometimes recommended high doses of vitamin C, up to 1,000 milligrams a day, for people with bladder or other urinary infections.

According to Mark Monane, M.D., an instructor at Harvard Medical School who was involved with the study, it wasn't the acidity of cranberries that helped keep bacteria in check. Rather, it appeared to be two compounds in the juice—fructose and a second compound yet to be identified—that helped prevent bacteria from adhering to the lining of the bladder and urethra.

Incidentally, Israeli researchers found that juice from blueberries—a close cousin of cranberries—had the same results.

In his book, *Doctor, What Should I Eat?*, Isadore Rosenfeld, M.D., clinical professor of medicine at New York Hospital–Cornell Medical Center in New York City, suggests women who have urinary tract infections drink two glasses (8 ounces each) of cranberry juice a day in addition to taking any antibiotics prescribed by their doctors. For women who are prone to infections and want to prevent them, drinking one glass every day will help ward off trouble.

# Getting the Most

**Eat them with relish.** Since raw cranberries contain considerably more healing compounds than cooked, you may want to try a cranberry relish. Put a pound of cranberries, two apples, and a large orange in a food processor and process until coarse. Mix in honey or sugar to taste, refrigerate for several hours, and serve.

**Have a drink.** Because raw cranberries have a tart taste and tough texture, you're unlikely to eat them raw. But you can still get the nutritional payload by drinking the juice.

Commercial cranberry juice cocktail drinks are loaded with vitamin C, with one glass containing a full day's supply. Unfortunately, most also have a full day's supply of sugar and are never more than 30 percent juice.

An alternative to supermarket juice is the juice found in health food stores. You can buy either pure cranberry juice or concentrated cranberry extract, which is used to make cold drinks or hot teas.

# Figs
## A FABULOUS FIBER FIND

Best known in this country for its role in the ever-popular Fig
Newton, the fig is perhaps the most significant fruit in history. The
Assyrians used figs as sweeteners as far back as 3000 B.C. Figs were
Cleopatra's favorite fruit. And some historians believe that figs, not
apples, were the forbidden fruit of the Garden of Eden—a debate that
may never be resolved, although certainly fig leaves were a convenient
fashion accessory of the time.

Today, we know that the fig is a fabulous source of fiber and a significant source of potassium. Plus, figs can add some hard-to-come-
by vitamin $B_6$ to your diet.

### FIGS AND FIBER

The average American gets only about 11 to 12 grams of dietary
fiber a day, far short of the 25 to 30 grams recommended by the American Dietetic Association. The Daily Value (DV) is 25 grams.

"Fiber is so good for so many things," says Diane Grabowski-Nepa,
R.D., a dietitian and nutritional counselor at the Pritikin Longevity
Center in Santa Monica, California. "Because fiber builds heavier
stools, it helps you eliminate waste more quickly and efficiently, which
studies show helps prevent constipation and colon cancer." Getting
more fiber in your diet also helps lower cholesterol and thus the risk
of heart disease.

Figs are an excellent source of fiber. Three figs, dried or fresh, provide about 5 grams of fiber, 20 percent of the DV. That 5 grams can
go a long way. A Harvard University study of 43,757 men ages 40 to
75 found that those who got the most fiber had about half the risk of
having heart attacks as those who got the least. Plus, men who added
just 10 grams of fiber a day to their diets dropped their risks of heart
disease by almost 30 percent.

"Figs are particularly good for people who are overweight, which is another risk for heart disease," says Grabowski-Nepa. Because they're so high in fiber, figs stay in the stomach longer, helping people eat less. "And they're very sweet, so they satisfy those sweet cravings," she adds.

## HELP FOR HIGH BLOOD PRESSURE

Figs are a good source of potassium, a mineral that's crucial for controlling blood pressure. Studies have shown that people who eat plenty of potassium-rich foods not only tend to have lower blood pressure but also have less risk of related conditions like stroke.

Potassium helps pull down high blood pressure in a number of ways. For one thing, it helps prevent dangerous low-density lipoprotein cholesterol from building up on artery walls, says David B. Young, Ph.D., professor of physiology and biophysics at the University of Mississippi Medical Center in Jackson. Plus, it helps remove excess sodium from inside cells, keeping the body's fluid levels in balance and blood pressure in check.

Three fresh figs contain 348 milligrams of potassium, 10 percent of the DV. Dried figs are even better, with three figs providing 399 milligrams, 11 percent of the DV.

## A BOOST OF $B_6$

Finally, figs can add some vitamin $B_6$ to your diet. While most of us get plenty of vitamin $B_6$, older people don't absorb it as efficiently as they once did. And since taking certain medications can also interfere with getting enough, getting extra amounts can be essential. Three fresh figs contain 0.18 milligram of $B_6$, 9 percent of the DV.

## Getting the Most

**Explore the sweetness.** One reason that people in this country don't eat a lot of figs is that they're not sure what to do with them. An easy way to get more of this fiber-rich food in your diet is to add it to foods that need a touch of sweetness, like cereals, cakes, or oatmeal. You can also mash figs into foods such as mashed potatoes. The fig's natural, nutty sweetness adds a great accent to mild foods while making it possible to eliminate flavorful but high-fat ingredients like butter or sour cream.

# Fish

## HEALTH FROM THE DEEP

For years, Americans have wisely been reducing the amount of fat in their diets. But there's one fat you may want to get more of: the fat in fish. When it comes to healthy eating, fish swims to first place.

Cold-water fish contain a number of polyunsaturated fats, which are known collectively as omega-3 fatty acids. Omega-3's benefit the fish by helping them stay warm in chilly waters. In people, the same fats go a long way toward promoting better health.

Consider Greenland's Eskimos. They eat fish to their hearts' content, which may be why they have very low levels of heart disease. Similar benefits have been observed around the world. People are simply a lot less likely to die from heart disease when fish plays a role in their diets.

"While further research is needed, there is compelling research that the oils in fish may contribute to controlling several conditions," says Gary J. Nelson, Ph.D., research chemist at the U.S. Department of Agriculture Western Human Nutrition Research Center in San Francisco. A diet high in fish, which helps block the production of potentially harmful chemicals in the body, does more than reduce the risk of heart disease. It also has been shown to help fight colon and breast cancers, promote larger-birthweight babies, and even reduce lung inflammation.

## SWIM AWAY FROM HEART DISEASE

In the 1980s, a round of studies reported that a diet high in fish could help protect against heart disease, prompting many Americans to trade some of their red meat and poultry for a couple of fish meals each week.

They made the right choice. Research has shown that people who eat fish are less likely to die from heart disease than their non-fish-eating counterparts. What's more, you don't have to eat a lot of fish to get the benefits. Evidence suggests that two fish meals a week is all you need to help keep your arteries open and your heart working well.

The omega-3's in fish appear to put the brakes on the body's production of prostaglandins, leukotrienes, and thromboxane, naturally occurring compounds that, in large amounts, may cause blood vessels to constrict, elevating blood pressure. These compounds also may promote unwanted clotting in the bloodstream, which can lead to heart disease.

The ability of omega-3's to prevent clotting is particularly important, says James Kenney, R.D., Ph.D., nutrition research specialist at the Pritikin Longevity Center in Santa Monica, California. Clots that form in the bloodstream can block the flow of blood to the heart, possibly causing heart attacks. Further, the oil found in fish appears to raise levels of high-density lipoprotein (HDL) cholesterol, the "good" cholesterol that helps keep fatty sludge from depositing in the arteries.

Research shows that fish can offer particular benefits to people who have already had one heart attack. Having two fish meals (each including about 3 ounces of fish) a week may reduce the chances of suffering a second, fatal heart attack. It also appears that eating more cold-water fish such as salmon may help keep arteries from closing after angioplasty, a procedure used to unclog blocked blood vessels in the heart.

In addition to its favorable effects on clotting and cholesterol, the oil in fish appears to help keep the heart beating in a healthy rhythm. This is important because potentially serious heartbeat irregularities, called arrhythmias, may lead to cardiac arrest, in which the heart stops beating entirely. There is increasing evidence that the omega-3's in fish somehow fortify the heart muscle and keep it beating regularly. In one study, people getting nearly 6 grams of omega-3's a month—the equivalent of having a 3-ounce serving of salmon weekly—had half the risk of cardiac arrest as those who ate no omega-3's.

While the benefits of adding more fish to your diet are well-known, you don't want to overdo it. One large study led by researchers at Northwestern University Medical School in Chicago found that those who ate more than 8 ounces of fish a week had higher stroke rates than those who ate less. This doesn't mean, however, that you should stop eating fish, says Dr. Kenney. Having small portions (2 to 3 ounces) twice a week will provide most of the benefits without the possible risks.

## STOPPING CANCER

Nutritionists have long advised us to eat less fat, especially the fats in meats and dairy products, to reduce the risk of certain types of cancer. But the fat in fish is a healthy exception. "There's excellent evidence that eating fish provides protection against breast and colorectal cancers," says Bandaru S. Reddy, Ph.D., chief of the division of nutritional carcinogenesis at the American Health Foundation in Valhalla, New York.

Fish protects against cancer in much the same way that it helps prevent heart disease—by reducing the body's production of prostaglandins. In large amounts, prostaglandins act as tumor promoters—that is, they encourage cancer tumors to grow, says Dr. Reddy.

In a study of people in 24 European countries, British researchers found that people who regularly included fish in their diets were much less likely to get cancer. Indeed, they estimated that having small servings of fish three times a week, in addition to decreasing intake of animal fats, would reduce the death rate from colon cancer in men by nearly one-third.

## BETTER BREATHING

You wouldn't think that eating fish could improve breathing difficulties caused by smoking, but that's exactly what researchers have found. People who smoke sometimes have a condition called chronic obstructive pulmonary disease, in which the ability to move oxygen in and out of the lungs is greatly reduced. There's some evidence that eating fish may help prevent this from occurring.

There's only so much that the occasional tuna steak can do to protect you from this disease if you smoke. But if you're trying to quit or if you live with someone who smokes, eating fish is one way to reduce the damage.

## MULTIPLE PROTECTION

Here are two additional reasons to get more fish in your diet. In one study, researchers looked at the fish-eating habits of more than 1,000 expectant moms in the Faeroe Islands, an area north of the United Kingdom. They found that the more fish the women ate, the larger their babies were likely to be. In fact, babies whose moms frequently had fish were, on average, nearly a half-pound heavier than those whose moms had less. This is important because larger babies are usually healthier than those who are underweight.

Researchers speculate that the omega-3's in fish help promote blood flow through the placenta, allowing the fetus to get more nutrients. In addition, by blocking the effects of prostaglandins, which are responsible for initiating uterine contractions, omega-3's might help prevent early labors and deliveries.

# Getting the Most

**Shop for salmon.** All fish provide some omega-3's, but salmon is perhaps the best choice, with a 3-ounce serving of Chinook salmon providing 3 grams.

**Look for deep colors.** The more deeply colored the salmon, the more omega-3's it provides. For example, Chinook salmon has the most oil, while the lighter pink salmon has a bit less. As a rule of thumb, the more expensive varieties of salmon generally have the most omega-3's.

**Shop for variety.** It's not only salmon that has omega-3's. Other good sources include mackerel, rainbow trout, tuna, whitefish (fresh, not smoked), and pickled Atlantic herring.

**Enjoy it canned.** One of the easiest way to get more omega-3's into your diet is to pick up a can of water-packed tuna. But if you're making tuna salad, be sure not to drown it in mayonnaise. The unhealthy fats in regular mayonnaise will more than offset the benefits of the healthy fats in the fish.

While you're in the canned food aisle, you may want to pick up a can of sardines, which also have good amounts of omega-3's.

**Use your microwave.** The high cooking temperatures used in conventional cooking methods such as broiling can destroy nearly half the omega-3's in fish. Microwaving has little effect on these beneficial oils, however, so it's a good cooking choice for getting the most benefits from your catch.

# Flaxseed

## GOOD FOR THE HEART—
## AND MORE

For centuries, flaxseed (and the plant from which it comes) was used for just about everything except food. Flax is one of the oldest sources of textile fiber and is used in making linen. Its seed, also known as linseed, is used for making paint. In the modern world, the closest it ever came to being a food was its use as a livestock feed.

Until recently, that is. Nowadays, because of its new-found fame as a "health food," Americans are enjoying the slightly sweet, nutty taste of flaxseed. And they're getting protection from heart disease and cancer as a reward.

### CANCER CONTROL

Flaxseed is an incredibly rich source of a group of compounds called lignans. While many plant foods also contain lignans, flaxseed has the absolute most—at least 75 times more than any other plant food. (You'd have to eat about 60 cups of fresh broccoli or 100 slices of whole-wheat bread to get the same amount of lignans that are in $1/4$ cup of flaxseed.) This is important because lignans may have powerful antioxidant properties that can help block the damaging effects of harmful oxygen molecules called free radicals. These molecules are thought to cause changes in the body that can lead to cancer.

"Lignans subdue cancerous changes once they've occurred, rendering them less likely to race out of control and develop into full-blown cancer," says flax researcher Lilian Thompson, Ph.D., professor of nutritional sciences at the University of Toronto.

Lignans show particular promise for battling breast cancer. They do this by blocking the effects of estrogen, which, over time, seems to increase breast cancer risk in some women. Even when estrogen-sensitive tumors get a chance to grow, lignans exert a restraining influence that can slow or even halt their growth. In a laboratory study, breast tumors in animals given flaxseed shrank by 50 percent in seven weeks.

Flaxseed has two additional cancer-fighting secrets. First, it is a rich source of polyunsaturated fats, including omega-3 fatty acids, which appear to limit the body's production of chemicals called prostaglandins. This is important because prostaglandins, in large amounts, can "speed up tumor growth," says Bandaru S. Reddy, Ph.D., chief of the division of nutritional carcinogenesis at the American Health Foundation in Valhalla, New York.

In addition, flaxseed is very high in fiber. Three tablespoons of seeds contains 3 grams of fiber, about 12 percent of the Daily Value. Fiber in the diet is very important because it can help block the effects of harmful compounds in the body that over time may cause damage to cells in the intestine and lead to cancer. It also moves these compounds out of the intestine more quickly, making them less likely to do harm.

## Heart and Kidney Helper

Some of the same compounds in flaxseed that battle cancer also show promise for reducing the risk of heart disease. Studies show that the omega-3's in flaxseed (which are also found in fish) appear to reduce blood clotting that can increase the risk of heart disease and stroke.

Flaxseed also appears to lower levels of dangerous low-density lipoprotein (LDL) cholesterol, the kind that contributes to heart disease. In one small study, people who ate 50 grams (about 5 tablespoons) of flaxseed a day for four weeks were able to reduce levels of harmful LDL cholesterol by up to 8 percent.

In addition, flaxseed shows promise for reversing kidney damage caused by lupus, a condition in which the immune system produces harmful substances that attack and damage healthy tissues. When researchers at the University of Western Ontario gave flaxseed to nine people with lupus-related kidney disease, they discovered that several measurements of kidney function, including the ability to filter waste, quickly improved.

The researchers speculate that the lignans and omega-3's in flaxseed fight inflammation in the tiny and very fragile arteries that supply blood to the kidneys, helping reduce the artery-clogging process that can lead to kidney damage.

Finally, laboratory research suggests that the lignans in flaxseed have bacteria- and fungus-fighting abilities, which means that it could be an aid in fighting infections.

## Getting the Most

**Buy it processed.** Many people sprinkle whole flaxseed on salads or fresh-baked breads. Flaxseed in this form provides little benefit, however, because the body is unable to crack open the hard little shells. So it's best to buy the cracked or milled forms, which readily give up the nutritious goodness packed inside.

**Pass on the oil.** Some manufacturers, in an attempt to capitalize on flaxseed's healthful reputation, are touting flaxseed oil as a source of omega-3's. Some are even offering high-lignan oil that contains some of the seed residue.

But don't spend your money just yet. There are good reasons to let the oil slide. Most of the lignans found in flaxseed are in the meal, which is the non-oil part of the seed. While the oil may contain some lignans, it can't compete with the seeds. In addition, while flaxseed oil isn't without benefits, it doesn't provide as much of the other healthful compounds found in the seeds, like fiber, protein, and minerals.

"Even though you might get the same amount of one health-promoting substance from the oil, it's better to go for the whole food," says Cindy Moore, R.D., director of nutrition therapy at the Cleveland Clinic Foundation in Ohio. "Chances are, you'll be getting other substances that you need for good health that researchers haven't even discovered yet."

# Garlic
## GREAT BULBS OF POWER

Filmmaker Les Blank made a documentary in 1980 called *Garlic Is as Good as 10 Mothers*. If he were to make a sequel today, he might call it *Garlic Is as Good as 1,200 Studies*.

An enormous amount of research has been done on this pungent bulb, and the results have been, quite literally, amazing. Dozens of medical benefits have been linked to garlic.

- Studies show that garlic lowers cholesterol and thins the blood, which may help prevent high blood pressure, heart disease, and stroke.
- In the laboratory, garlic appears to block the growth of cancer cells. Population studies show that people who eat lots of garlic have fewer stomach and colon cancers than those who eat the least.
- In a study at Boston City Hospital, garlic was successfully used to kill 14 strains of bacteria taken from the noses and throats of children with ear infections.

In addition, research has shown that garlic can help boost immunity and reduce high levels of blood sugar. It may also relieve asthma and keep individual cells healthy and strong, perhaps delaying or preventing some of the conditions associated with aging.

Garlic's healing potential has been recognized for thousands of years. Historically, it's been used to treat everything from wounds and infections to digestion problems. In World War II, for example, when Russian soldiers ran out of penicillin for their wounds, they requisitioned garlic cloves. And today, in Germany, Japan, and other modern countries, garlic formulas are sold as over-the-counter drugs.

## GOOD FOR THE HEART
Thus far, researchers have identified two important ways in which garlic is good for the heart and circulation. First, it contains many

sulfur compounds, including diallyl disulfide (DADS), which seem to smooth blood flow by helping to prevent platelets from sticking together and clotting. In a study at Brown University in providence, Rhode Isalnd, researchers gave 45 men with high cholesterol aged garlic extract—about the equivalent of five to six cloves of fresh garlic. When they examined the men's blood, they saw that the rate at which platelets clumped and stuck together had dropped anywhere from 10 to 58 percent.

"High platelet activity means that you're more likely to have arteriosclerosis or a heart attack or a stroke," says researcher Robert I. Lin, Ph.D., executive vice president of Nutrition International in Irvine, California. "But sulfur compounds are very potent. They thin the blood."

Garlic is also good for the heart because it lowers the levels of cholesterol and blood fats called triglycerides in the bloodstream. According to Yu-Yan Yeh, Ph.D., professor of nutrition science at Pennsylvania State University in University Park, many of garlic's protective effects take place in the liver, where cholesterol is produced. In laboratory studies, rats given garlic extract produced 87 percent less cholesterol and 64 percent fewer trigylcerides.

"The liver is a primary place in the body for fat synthesis and for production of blood cholesterol," says Dr. Yeh. "When fewer of these substances are made in the liver, there are fewer of them in the blood."

In a review of 16 studies involving 952 people, British researchers found that eating garlic—whether fresh or in powdered form—lowered total cholesterol an average of 12 to 13 percent. And according to a review by researchers at New York Medical College in Valhalla, scientific evidence suggests that eating one-half to one clove of garlic daily could reduce blood cholesterol levels by about 9 percent.

## CANCER PROTECTION

There's increasing evidence that including garlic in the diet may play a role in preventing and treating cancer. Studies suggest that garlic can help block cancer in several ways: by preventing cell changes that lead to cancer, by stopping tumors from growing, or by killing the harmful cells outright.

• A compound in garlic called s-allylcysteine appears to stop the metabolic action that causes a healthy cell to become cancerous, says John Milner, Ph.D., professor and head of the department of nutrition at Pennsylvania State University.

• The substance called DADS, which we discussed earlier, appears to throttle the growth of cancer cells by interfering with their ability to divide and multiply. "DADS chokes cancer cells until their numbers are reduced and they start dying," says Dr. Milner.

• Another substance in garlic is diallyl trisulfide (DATS), which is 10 times more powerful than DADS at killing human lung cancer cells. "Its effectiveness is comparable to that of 5-fluorouracil, a widely used chemotherapy agent," Dr. Milner says. And since garlic is vastly less toxic to healthy cells than the chemotherapy drug, there's hope that some day garlic could form the basis for a gentler chemotherapy.

• Garlic contains compounds that help prevent nitrites—common substances found in some foods as well as a variety of everyday pollutants—from transforming themselves into nitrosamines, harmful compounds that can trigger cancerous changes in the body.

Garlic's benefits aren't seen only in the laboratory. For example, researchers have noted that people in Southern Italy, who eat a lot of garlic, develop less stomach cancer than the non-garlic-eaters to their north.

"In one province of northern China, people routinely eat four to seven cloves of garlic a day. For every 100 cases of stomach cancer in the neighboring province, where garlic intake isn't as high, the garlic-eating population will suffer eight or fewer cases," says Dr. Paxton.

Closer to home, a study of 41,837 women living in Iowa found that those who ate garlic at least once a week had a 35 percent lower risk of colon cancer than women who never ate garlic.

"If I had to take an educated guess, I'd say that eating three cloves of garlic a day might reduce your risk of many cancers by 20 percent," says Dr. Lin. "And eating six cloves could get you at least a 30 percent reduction," he adds.

## WELCOME "GARLICILLIN"

A frightening trend in recent years has been antibiotic resistance—the ability of bacteria to shrug off the effects of once-effective drugs. Recent research suggests garlic may be effective where traditional drugs have failed or are too toxic.

In one study, researchers at Boston City Hospital swabbed 14 different strains of bacteria from the noses and throats of children with ear infections. Some of the infections had been impervious to treatment with antibiotics. In the laboratory, however, garlic extract effectively killed the resistant germs.

In another study, researchers at the University of New Mexico, Albuquerque, tested whether garlic could be used to treat otomycosis, or swimmer's ear. Swimmer's ear is caused, scientists think, by a fungus called aspergillus. And normal treatments for it are less than ideal. Topical drugs can be uncomfortable and cannot be used if the ear drum has already been broken.

In the laboratory study, researchers treated swimmer's ear fungi with a mixture of garlic extract and water. Even at very low concentrations, the garlic blocked the growth of fungi just as well as available drugs. And, in some cases, it proved even better.

# Getting the Most

**Enjoy it fresh.** Crushed raw garlic contains allicin, a compound that breaks down quickly into a cascade of healthful compounds, like DADS and DATS. Of course, not everyone enjoys the bite of raw garlic. Try cutting a clove in half and rubbing it hard against the inside of a wooden salad bowl before putting in the salad. You'll get just a hint of garlic taste and more than a hint of garlic benefits.

**But eat for convenience.** You don't have to prepare fresh garlic to get the healing benefits; each form of garlic—raw, cooked, or powdered—has its own important compounds. By taking advantage of each of these forms, you can slip more garlic and its healing compounds into your menu.

**Cut it fine.** Whether you're cooking garlic or eating it raw, mincing, crushing, or pressing it vastly expands the surface area, maximizing the production and release of healthful compounds.

**Cook it lightly.** Overcooking garlic can destroy some of the delicate compounds. It's best to cook it lightly—stir-fried with vegetables, for example, or added to a long-cooking stew in the last few minutes of cooking time—suggests Dr. Lin. "The taste is much more gentle than raw garlic," he says.

# Ginger
## THE PUNGENT HEALER

$R$oman doctors kept it handy during military marches. Pythagoras, Greek philosopher and geometry whiz, touted it for digestive health. And King Henry VIII of England was convinced that it would protect against plague, although there's no evidence that ginger is that good. But there's plenty of evidence that this gnarled, piquant root can help relieve dozens of conditions, from motion sickness and other digestive complaints to migraines, arthritis, high cholesterol, and even dangerous blood clots. This is why millions of people worldwide swear by ginger as a potent healing food.

### HELP FOR THE HEAVES

As anyone who has experienced motion sickness knows, even a mild bout can derail the best-laid vacation plans. That's why nearly every travel checklist, along with reminders to buy sunscreen and feed the cat, includes the notation, "Buy Dramamine."

The next time you travel, you may want to stop at the supermarket instead of the pharmacy. As it turns out, ginger is one of the best motion sickness remedies you can buy.

In a classic study conducted by Daniel B. Mowrey, Ph.D., director of the American Phytotherapy Research Laboratory in Salt Lake City, 36 motion sickness–prone students were strapped into tilted rotating chairs and spun until they felt ill. Those who were given 100 milligrams of dimenhydrinate (Dramamine) beforehand couldn't take the stomach-churning ride for more than about $4^1/_2$ minutes, and most gave up sooner. Half of those given ginger, however, were able to withstand the ride for the full 6 minutes, with less nausea and dizziness than the drug-treated group.

In another study, Dutch researchers testing the effects of ginger on seasick naval cadets found that ginger pills reduced the cadets' nausea and vomiting, providing relief for as long as 4 hours.

Experts aren't sure why ginger suppresses a queasy stomach. But researchers in Japan have suggested that gingerols, one of the active ingredients in ginger, may be indirectly responsible for blocking the body's vomiting reflex.

To use ginger for combating motion sickness, take about $1/4$ teaspoon of fresh or powdered ginger 20 minutes before getting in a car or on a boat, advises Varro E. Tyler, Ph.D., professor emeritus of pharmacognosy at Purdue University School of Pharmacy in West Lafayette, Indiana. Repeat every few hours as needed.

You can also use ginger to help relieve a run-of-the-mill upset stomach. Prepare a cup of ginger tea by adding three or four thin slices of fresh ginger to a cup of boiling water, and sip as needed, advises Charles Lo, M.D., a doctor of Chinese medicine in private practice in Chicago.

## RELIEF FOR MIGRAINES

If you're one of the millions of Americans who suffer from migraine headaches, ginger may help keep the pain and nausea away. In a small study, researchers at Odense University in Denmark found that ginger may short-circuit impending migraines without the bothersome side effects of some migraine-relieving drugs. It appears that ginger blocks the action of prostaglandins, substances that cause pain and inflammation in blood vessels in the brain.

Research is still very preliminary, so experts are reluctant to recommend specific treatment plans for using ginger to fight migraines. If you feel a headache coming on, you may want to try taking $1/3$ teaspoon of fresh or powdered ginger, which is the amount suggested by the Danish researchers.

## AID FOR ARTHRITIS

Are the joints in your fingers so stiff and sore that you can't fumble the childproof cap off the aspirin bottle? You may want to add ginger to your medicine chest.

In one study, Danish researchers studied 56 people who had either rheumatoid arthritis or osteoarthritis and who treated themselves with fresh or powdered ginger. They found that ginger produced "marked" relief in 55 percent of people with osteoarthritis and 74 percent of those with rheumatoid arthritis.

Some experts speculate that ginger may ease arthritis pain the same way it helps block migraines, by blocking the formation of inflammation-causing prostaglandins that cause pain and swelling.

To soothe arthritis pain, Dr. Lo recommends brewing a mild tea, again, by putting three or four slices of fresh ginger in a cup of boiling water. You can also try taking $1/2$ teaspoon of powdered ginger or up to an ounce (about 6 teaspoons) of fresh ginger once a day, which are the amounts consumed by people in the Danish arthritis study.

## HELP FOR THE BLOOD

Blood clots can be a good thing. When you cut your finger, for example, platelets—components in blood that help it clot—help "stick" the wound together so that it can heal.

But these sticky platelets can also cling to artery walls and to each other. When that happens, clots stop being beneficial and become something to worry about. Many people routinely take aspirin to help keep their blood clear of clots that could lead to strokes or heart attacks.

It turns out that ginger may do a little bit of the same thing. In an unusual incident at Cornell University Medical College in New York City, a researcher working with his own blood noticed that it wasn't clotting as it usually did. Eventually, he remembered the large amount of ginger marmalade that he had eaten the previous day. On a hunch, he mixed platelets from his blood with powdered ginger. Sure enough, clotting was inhibited.

The gingerol in ginger has a chemical structure somewhat similar to that of aspirin. Research suggests that getting ginger in the diet—although at this point, experts aren't sure how much—may inhibit the production of a chemical called thromboxane, which plays a key role in the clotting process.

A last word about blood: Studies have shown that ginger, both fresh and powdered, may help lower cholesterol. Researchers in India fed laboratory animals various mixtures of spices, including ginger. They found that ginger, and also red pepper and mustard, helped speed the conversion of cholesterol to bile acids, which is the body's way of removing excess cholesterol before it does harm.

# Getting the Most

**Use it fresh.** Ginger comes in a variety of forms, including fresh, dried, crystallized, and powdered. It's best to use it fresh, advises Dr. Lo. "Fresh ginger is more active than dried," he says. Crystallized ginger is almost as good, he adds.

At the grocery store, try to buy the freshest ginger to get the most healing compounds. "Avoid ginger with soft spots, mold, or dry, wrinkled skin," Dr. Lo advises.

**Use a grater.** Grating fresh ginger releases more of its potent juice than slicing or chopping, says Dr. Lo. Using a garlic press will also extract the maximum amount of juice from the root.

**Enjoy it often.** To squeeze the most health benefits from ginger, consume it as often as possible, says Dr. Lo. But you don't need to go ginger-crazy to get the healing benefits. Less than an ounce a day will do. "Drinking a few cups of ginger tea or adding a small amount of fresh ginger to a stir-fry should be enough."

**Choose the right root.** Whenever possible, buy ginger grown in Africa or India, says Stephen Fulder, Ph.D., a private research consultant and author of *The Ginger Book*. Studies show that these varieties are more potent than the common Jamaican kind.

You can't tell the difference in gingers just by looking, though. Ask the produce manager at the supermarket or health food store. He should be able to tell you which variety he's selling.

# Greens

## NATURE'S BEST PROTECTION

Double coupons, good gas mileage, blue-light specials—if there's one thing that Americans appreciate, it's getting more for less.

That is why we really ought to love leafy green vegetables. They deliver more nutrients for fewer calories than virtually any food out there.

"You get so many important nutrients from leafy green vegetables—magnesium, iron, calcium, folate, vitamin C, and vitamin $B_6$, plus all the heart disease– and cancer-fighting phytochemicals," says Michael Liebman, Ph.D., professor of human nutrition at the University of Wyoming in Laramie. "These are the most nutrient-dense foods that we have available."

Experts are quick to note, however, that American's favorite "salad starter"—the bland-tasting iceberg lettuce—doesn't count as a "leafy green" vegetable. Of all the foods in this powerhouse family, iceberg is the runt. Far better are such things as kale, Swiss chard, dandelion greens, beet greens, mustard greens, turnip greens, spinach, and chicory greens.

### LEAVES FOR THE HEART

To some extent, the difference between people who have heart attacks and those who don't may be how many trips they make to the salad bar.

Researchers from the Jean Mayer USDA Human Nutrition Research Center on Aging at Tufts University in Boston and the Framingham Heart Study in Massachusetts studied more than 1,000 people between the ages of 67 and 95 to learn what dietary factors affect heart health. In this, as in so many issues touching on food, the answer boiled down to chemistry—specifically, to an amino acid called homocysteine.

Homocysteine is a natural compound that is harmless as long as the body keeps it in check. When it reaches high levels, however, it becomes toxic and may contribute to clogged arteries and heart disease. The researchers found that among people with the most clogged arteries, 43 percent of men and 34 percent of women had high levels of homocysteine in their blood.

What's the connection with greens? The body uses folate and vitamins $B_{12}$ and $B_6$ to keep homocysteine under control. Many of the people in the study were falling short of these vital nutrients—especially folate and vitamin $B_6$.

As it turns out, leafy greens are outstanding sources of folate, and they also provide vitamin $B_6$. That's why experts advise adding plenty of leafy green vegetables to your diet to counteract homocysteine levels.

Boiled spinach is probably your best bet. A half-cup of Popeye's favorite snack delivers 131 micrograms of folate, 33 percent of the Daily Value (DV). It also contains 0.2 milligram of vitamin $B_6$, 10 percent of the DV.

In addition to these important B vitamins, certain greens—particularly beet greens, chicory, and spinach—provide the heart-healthy minerals magnesium, potassium, and calcium. These minerals, along with sodium, help regulate the amount of fluid that your body retains. All too often, researchers say, people have too much sodium and too little of the other three, leading to high blood pressure.

Even though eating leafy greens is an excellent way to help regulate blood pressure, it's important to note that the calcium from spinach and beet greens isn't well-absorbed by the body. Be sure to eat a wide variety of greens to meet all your mineral needs.

## MEAT OF THE DIET

Large studies overwhelmingly show that cancers of the lung, esophagus, colon, head, and neck occur least often in countries where people regard leafy greens, along with a wide variety of fruits and vegetables, as the "meats" of their meals.

In one study, researchers compared 61 men with lung cancer in Chile with 61 men of similar age and smoking habits who were cancer-free. The one difference they found was that men with cancer consumed significantly fewer carotenoid-rich foods, especially Swiss chard, chicory, and spinach as well as beets and cabbage, than those without the disease.

The carotenoids, which are found in large amounts in most leafy greens, are like bodyguards against cancer-causing agents, explains Frederick Khachik, Ph.D., research chemist at the Food Composition Laboratory at the U.S. Department of Agriculture in Beltsville, Maryland. Scientists believe that certain cancers are brought on by the constant onslaught of free radicals—harmful oxygen molecules made by our bodies and also found in air pollution and tobacco smoke—which attack our bodies' healthy cells. Carotenoids counteract free radicals by acting as antioxidants, meaning that they step between the free radicals and our bodies' cells, neutralizing them before they can do damage, he explains.

"There is also plenty of evidence that carotenoids may fight cancer by activating the body's detoxification enzymes—called phase II enzymes—which are responsible for ridding the body of harmful, often cancer-causing chemicals," says Dr. Khachik.

"Dark green, leafy vegetables are among the best sources of some very important carotenoids, like lutein, alpha-carotene, and the one that everyone's familiar with, beta-carotene," he says.

While all leafy greens are rich in carotenoids, the granddaddy is spinach, with a half-cup providing 1 milligram of beta-carotene. When the beta-carotene is converted into vitamin A in the body, it delivers 37 percent of the DV for vitamin A.

## SEEING GREEN

Carrots must be good for your eyes, the old joke has it, since you never see a rabbit wearing glasses. According to research, it's probably not only carrots that are good for the eyes but also all the leafy greens that Peter and his cotton-tailed friends munch.

In one study, scientists from the Massachusetts Eye and Ear Infirmary in Boston compared the diets of more than 350 people with advanced age-related macular degeneration—the leading cause of irreversible vision loss among older adults—with the diets of more than 500 people without the disease. They found that people who ate the most leafy green vegetables—particularly spinach and collard greens—were 43 percent less likely to get macular degeneration than those who ate them less frequently.

Experts believe that carotenoids protect the eyes in much the same way as they work against cancer, by acting as antioxidants and neutralizing tissue-damaging free radicals before they harm the body—in this case, the macular region of the eye.

## SMILE AND SAY "GREENS"

In some parts of the world, like rural China, where vegetarianism is a way of life, people meet their daily calcium needs not by drinking milk but by eating greens.

In fact, 1 cup of turnip or dandelion greens can deliver about 172 milligrams of calcium, 17 percent of the DV. That's more than you'd get from a half-cup of skim milk.

The only problem with getting calcium from leafy green vegetables is that some of them contain high amounts of oxalates—compounds that block calcium absorption, says Dr. Liebman. "Spinach, Swiss chard, collards, and beet greens have the most oxalates, so don't consider these a source of calcium," he says. "The others are fine. Research has shown that the calcium in kale is particularly well-absorbed."

## PUMPING UP AT THE SALAD BAR

If you're among the many folks cutting back on meat these days, you may be cutting down on a very important mineral—iron—as well. Here again, the leafy greens can help. Many vegetables, especially spinach and Swiss chard, are good sources of iron, a mineral your body needs to produce red blood cells and transport oxygen.

A half-cup of boiled spinach has 3 milligrams of iron, 20 percent of the Recommended Dietary Allowance (RDA) for women and 30 percent of the RDA for men. The same amount of Swiss chard provides 2 milligrams, 13 percent of the RDA for women and 30 percent of the RDA for men.

Unfortunately, the iron found in plants isn't as readily absorbed by the body as the iron found in meats—unless it's accompanied in the same meal by vitamin C. Good news again. Along with their high doses of iron, leafy green vegetables also contain ample amounts of vitamin C, which substantially improves iron absorption.

Of course, vitamin C is also good in its own right—for fighting infections, like colds and flu, and for healing wounds. And like beta-carotene, vitamin C is an antioxidant, so it helps protect your body's cells from internal damage.

All the leafy greens provide ample amounts of this important nutrient, but the green giants of vitamin C are chicory (a half-cup serving has 22 milligrams, 37 percent of the DV) and beet and mustard greens, both providing almost 18 milligrams, 30 percent of the DV.

In addition, beet greens and spinach are rich sources of riboflavin—a B vitamin that is essential for tissue growth and repair as well as helping your body convert other nutrients into usable forms. A half-cup of cooked spinach or beet greens provides 0.2 milligram of riboflavin, 12 percent of the DV. Seeking riboflavin from plant sources like leafy green vegetables is especially important for people who avoid dairy products, which are among the best sources of these important nutrients.

# Getting the Most

**Cook them quickly.** To cook or not to cook? That's often the question asked by people who want to maintain the highest levels of healing nutrients in their vegetables. The answer with leafy greens, experts say, is yes, no, and maybe a little.

"It's always a trade-off between increasing the digestibility of nutrients when you cook foods and losing some nutrients in the cooking process," says Dr. Liebman. "But while it's great to eat them raw, you're more likely to eat more of certain vegetables if they're cooked. Just watch your cooking method. You don't want to boil them to death. Any quick-cooking method, such as blanching, is fine. One of the best cooking methods for retaining nutrients seems to be the microwave," he says.

# Honey

## THE BEST FROM THE BEES

In Greek mythology, the infant Zeus was kept alive by bees that fed him honey while he was hidden away in a cave, and he was so grateful that he rewarded the bees by giving them high intelligence.

Even today, when sugary foods are hardly in short supply, there's something special about honey. Not only is it sweeter, ounce for ounce, than table sugar, but its wonderfully thick, liquid texture makes it a natural for spreading on cakes, crackers, and breads.

Although honey contains trace amounts of minerals and B vitamins, it's really not much more nutritious than plain table sugar. Yet honey does several things that sugar doesn't. "Some people have called honey a remedy rediscovered," says Peter Molan, Ph.D., professor of biochemistry and director of the Honey Research Unit at the University of Waikato in Hamilton, New Zealand, who has been studying the healing properties of honey for 15 years.

## QUICKER HEALING

If you saw a jar of honey in your doctor's black bag, you'd just assume that he packed in the dark. But as it turns out, doctors have been using honey for centuries. Honey contains three ingredients that make it ideal for treating wounds. Because it's very high in sugar, it absorbs much of the moisture inside wounds, making it hard for bacteria to survive, Dr. Molan explains. In addition, many honeys contain large amounts of hydrogen peroxide, the same medicine you use at home to disinfect cuts and scrapes. Finally, some honeys contain propolis, a compound in nectar that can kill bacteria.

In a laboratory study, Dr. Molan smeared honey on seven types of bacteria that often cause wound infections. "It very effectively killed all seven types," he says.

## Sweetness Within

Just as honey can stop infections on the outside of your body, it also can keep you healthy on the inside. A type of honey called Manuka, for example, which is produced when bees feed on a type of flowering shrub in New Zealand, appears to kill the bacteria that cause stomach ulcers. In one small study, people with ulcers were given 1 tablespoon of Manuka honey four times a day. "The honey relieved ulcer symptoms in all the people who took it," Dr. Molan says.

Honey also shows promise for treating diarrhea. In children particularly, diarrhea can be dangerous because it removes large amounts of water from the body. To replace fluids and essential minerals, doctors have traditionally treated diarrhea with a sugar solution. But a honey solution may be even better because honey can kill intestinal bacterial that may be causing the problem. In fact, researchers at the University of Natal in South Africa found that when children with diarrhea caused by a bacterial infection were given a honey solution, they got better in almost half the time of those who were given a traditional sugar solution.

Honey may work against constipation as well. It contains large amounts of fructose, a sugar that sometimes arrives in the large intestine undigested. When bacteria in the intestine begin the process of fermentation, water is drawn into the bowel, which acts as a laxative, explains Marvin Schuster, M.D., director of the Marvin M. Schuster Digestive and Motility Disorders Center at Johns Hopkins Bayview Medical Center in Baltimore. Honey is higher in fructose than just about any other food, he adds.

# Getting the Most

**Shop for raw honey.** The high heats used in making processed honey will disable some of the protective compounds, says Dr. Molan. To get the most antibacterial power, raw honey is your best bet.

**Make it Manuka.** While most raw honeys contain some active ingredients, Manuka honey contains the most. This is particularly important when you're taking honey for relieving ulcers, Dr. Molan says. You can often find Manuka honey in health food stores. It's important, however, to read the label to make sure you're getting "active Manuka honey." If it doesn't contain the active compounds, it won't be effective for ulcers, Dr. Molan says.

# Lemons
# and Limes

## PUCKER POWER

You may love the tartness of lemons and limes, but it's a good bet that you've never taken a big bite from the whole fruit. Back in the nineteenth century, however, people literally craved them, not for their tart blast but for their remarkable health benefits.

British sailors, for example, would quaff lime juice to prevent scurvy, a terrible disease caused by vitamin C deficiency. (It was because of the British Navy's dependence on limes that they became known as limeys.) And in California during the Gold Rush, when fresh fruits were equally scarce, miners paid top dollar for lemons.

## A SEA OF C

Of all the nutrients we're most familiar with, vitamin C is perhaps the most impressive. During cold season it's always in hot demand, since it lowers levels of histamine, a naturally occurring chemical that can cause red eyes and runny noses. Vitamin C is also a powerful antioxidant, meaning that it helps disarm powerful oxygen molecules in the body that contribute to cancer and heart disease. The body also uses vitamin C to manufacture collagen, the stuff that glues cells together and is needed to help heal cuts and wounds.

The pulp and juice from lemons and limes are rich sources of vitamin C. A large lemon, for example, contains about 45 milligrams of vitamin C, 75 percent of the Daily Value (DV). Limes are also good, with a small lime containing about 20 milligrams, 33 percent of the DV.

Of course, unless you have an asbestos tongue and an astonishing passion for tartness, you're not likely to eat a whole lemon or lime every day. But squeezing a little juice on your salad or fish or pouring a tall glass of sweetened fresh-squeezed juice will help boost your levels of this important nutrient.

## QUEST FOR THE ZEST

There's more to lemons and limes than vitamin C. They contain additional compounds such as limonin and limonene, which appear to help block some of the cellular changes that can lead to cancer.

Limonene, which is found mainly in the colorful skin, or zest, of the fruit, has been shown to increase the activity of proteins that help eliminate estradiol, a naturally occurring hormone that has been linked with breast cancer. Limonene has also been shown to increase the level of enzymes in the liver that can remove cancer-causing chemicals.

In Europe, food companies add citrus zest to baking flour for the added health benefits, says Antonio Montanari, Ph.D., research scientist with the Florida Department of Citrus Research Center in Lake Alfred. "Here in America, we throw away what may be the best part of the fruit," he says.

# Getting the Most

**Zest up your flavors.** Whether you're making a lemon meringue pie or simply adding flavor to store-bought lemon yogurt, be sure to add plenty of zest. The healing compound limonene makes up about 65 percent of oils in the peel, says Michael Gould, Ph.D., professor of human oncology at the University of Wisconsin Medical School in Madison.

**Use it dried.** While fresh citrus peel contains the most healing compounds, dried lemon peel isn't bad, says Dr. Montanari. You'll find dried lemon peel in the spice rack at the supermarket.

**Enjoy it juiced.** Since lemons and limes are so tart, sweet lemonade is about the only way to get large amounts of them into your diet. Many people prefer using canned concentrate because it's convenient and it retains many of the healthful compounds. Fresh juice is even better. Simply squeeze your lemons or limes and add sugar or honey to sweeten. Adding a little zest from the peel will give the juice a pleasant taste and put more limonene into the mix.

**Let the two tango.** To add a slightly exotic, Caribbean twist to lemonade, try adding a little lime juice. You can use fresh or bottled, although the fresh juice has a third more vitamin C than the bottled kind.

# Melons

## HEALTH FROM THE VINE

Summer picnics don't really come alive until the barbecue is cold and the potato salad has been put away. That's when it's time to pick up a knife and cut into the tough green rind of an ice-cold watermelon, revealing the sweet red flesh within.

There's always something exciting about cutting open a watermelon, crenshaw, or honeydew. For one thing, they come encased in protective rinds, so what's inside always comes as a surprise. And even before you cut, most melons whet your appetite by releasing a rich, penetrating scent, which is why they're sometimes called the "perfumy fruits."

Here's another reason melons are so marvelous. Researchers have found that they contain a number of substances that are very good for your health. Both watermelons and muskmelons—which include honeydews, crenshaws, and a few other melons—provide folate, a B vitamin that has been shown to lower the risks of birth defects and heart disease. Melons also contain potassium, which is essential for keeping blood pressure at healthy levels. And because melons are low in calories and fat, they're the perfect food for waist-watchers.

### MELONS FOR MOMS—AND MORE

Folate has a less-than-illustrious history. For a long time, doctors weren't sure what folate did. They suspected that it played a role in preventing birth defects, but there wasn't strong evidence one way or the other. Then a study of almost 4,000 mothers revealed that those who got enough folate were 60 percent less likely to have children with brain and spinal cord defects (called neural tube defects) than women who got smaller amounts.

So before you start shopping for pickles, put a few melons in your cart because they're very good sources of folate. A cup of honeydew, for example, contains 11 micrograms of folate, 3 percent of the Daily Value (DV). Casaba melons are even better, with the same cup providing 29 micrograms of folate, 7 percent of the DV.

If 7 percent doesn't sound like a lot, remember that a cup of melon is the equivalent of about five good bites. Most people eat two or more cups of melon at a time, making it a very good folate find.

Incidentally, it's not only moms-to-be who should be making the most of melons. The same nutrient that protects against birth defects is also good for the heart.

The body uses folate to control levels of a chemical in the blood called homocysteine. "Although small amounts of homocysteine are normal, too much of it somehow contributes to the artery-clogging process that leads to heart disease," says Killian Robinson, M.D., a cardiologist at the Cleveland Clinic Foundation in Ohio. "We know that low levels of folate are related to too-high homocysteine levels."

Finally, folate has been shown to reduce the risk of polyps, precancerous growths in the colon that sometimes progress to full-blown cancer. Researchers at Harvard Medical School found that people getting the most folate were 33 percent less likely to develop polyps in the colon than those getting the least.

## THE FIBER FIX

The one thing that your digestive tract needs more than almost anything else is a steady supply of dietary fiber. Fiber is so important, in fact, that people who don't get enough have higher risks for cancer as well as for a variety of digestive problems, says John H. Weisburger, Ph.D., senior member of the American Health Foundation in Valhalla, New York.

The type of fiber found in melons, called soluble fiber, is tremendously important for keeping the colon healthy, Dr. Weisburger explains. Because soluble fiber absorbs water as it move through the digestive tract, it causes stools to get heavier and larger. As a result, they move more quickly through the intestine, reducing the amount of time that harmful substances in the stool are in contact with the colon wall.

"Getting more fiber has been shown to reduce the number of polyps in the gastrointestinal tract and also the risk of colon cancer," says Dr. Weisburger. All melons contain some fiber, although honeydews beat out watermelon by quite a bit. Half a honeydew has nearly 3 grams of fiber, 12 percent of the DV.

## More Melons, Less Pressure

If you have high blood pressure, you're probably already getting less salt and more minerals in your diet. It's a good idea to get more melons as well. All melons, especially honeydews and crenshaws, are good sources of potassium, which is perhaps the most important mineral for keeping blood pressure down.

The potassium in melons acts as a natural diuretic, removing excess fluids from the body. This is important because when fluid levels are high, blood pressure can rise, says Michael T. Murray, a naturopathic doctor in Bellevue, Washington, and author of *Natural Alternatives to Over-the-Counter and Prescription Drugs*. Plus, potassium keeps the artery walls relaxed, which also helps keep blood pressure down.

People with high blood pressure are often advised to get at least the DV of 3,500 milligrams of potassium a day. Melons make it easy. Half a honeydew, for example, has about 1,355 milligrams of potassium, over a third of the DV. Watermelons also contain potassium, but only about half as much as honeydews or crenshaws.

# Getting the Most

**Make it a honey.** Even though watermelon is a decent source of nutrients, it contains so much water that they're very diluted. Ounce for ounce, honeydews have over twice the potassium and almost three times more folate than watermelon.

**Buy them whole.** Supermarkets often sell watermelons, honeydews, and other melons cut into halves or slices. This can save space in your refrigerator, but it won't save much in the way of nutrients. When the flesh of melons is exposed to light, the nutrients start to break down. So it's a good idea to buy melons whole. And once you've cut them, keep them covered in the refrigerator to prevent the vitamins from breaking down.

**Keep them cold.** Folate is readily destroyed by heat, so it's important to store melons, whole or cut, in a cool, dark place.

# Milk

## A Glassful of Goodness

Even people who love milk often feel guilty about indulging. Despite its old-time reputation as being the perfect food, milk is extremely high in fat. A cup of whole milk is 49 percent fat. Reduced-fat milk isn't much better. It contains 34 percent fat. Worse, most of this fat is saturated, the kind that clogs your arteries. Not exactly what you'd call "perfect."

Before you wipe away your milk mustache forever, consider the lighter side: low-fat and skim milk. A cup of low-fat milk gets only 23 percent of its calories from fat. Skim milk (also called nonfat or fat-free) is the ultimate, with virtually zero fat. Both skim and low-fat are two of the cheapest, easiest ways to help fulfill your daily requirements of a variety of important nutrients. Best of all, skim milk isn't the thin, gray, watery stuff it used to be. Several manufacturers, wise to the fact that consumers want the flavor of fat without the fat itself, now offer richer, creamier skims. Chances are, you won't be able to tell the difference.

"Once you get the fat out, milk is a highly nutritious food," says Curtis Mettlin, Ph.D., chief of epidemiologic research at Roswell Park Cancer Institute in Buffalo, New York. The many nutrients that milk contains can go a long way toward preventing high blood pressure, stroke, osteoporosis, and maybe even cancer—all for 85 calories, less than 5 grams of cholesterol, and less than 1 gram of fat per glassful of skim milk.

### Skim Past Heart Disease

If you're concerned about cholesterol, you're probably already eating foods like apples, oats, and beans. Milk, as it turns out, is another food that can send cholesterol south.

Researchers at Kansas State University in Manhattan, Kansas, and

Pennsylvania State University in University Park had 64 people drink a quart of skim milk a day. After a month, the people with the highest cholesterol levels saw their cholesterol drop almost 10 points. That's almost a 7-percent reduction. Since every 1-percent drop in cholesterol translates into a 2-percent reduction in death from heart disease, drinking milk helped these folks reduce their risks of heart attacks or strokes by nearly 14 percent.

"Studies have shown that milk contains substances that reduce the liver's production of cholesterol," says Arun Kilara, Ph.D., professor of food science at Pennsylvania State University and one of the researchers on the study.

Here's another great thing about milk. Its abundance of calcium may help reduce blood pressure as well as cholesterol. In the University Park study, drinking milk was able to lower systolic blood pressure (the top number), on average, from 131.1 to 126.4 after eight weeks, while diastolic pressure (the bottom number) dropped from 82.6 to 78.1.

Researchers aren't sure how much milk you should drink when trying to lower cholesterol or blood pressure. However, a good place to start would be with four glasses a day—the amount used in the study. If you think that's a lot, try drinking an 8-ounce glass of skim milk with each meal, then have one as a snack.

## THE BEST BONE-BUILDER

Milk is best known for its ability to help strengthen bones. There's good reason for this. Milk is an excellent source of calcium, with 1 cup skim containing more than 300 milligrams, almost a third of the Daily Value (DV). That's why drinking milk is often recommended as a great strategy for preventing osteoporosis, the bone-thinning disease that affects more than 28 million people in the United States, most of them women.

In a study of 581 women past menopause, researchers at the University of California, San Diego, found that those who drank the most milk in their teens and early 20s had stronger bones than those who drank less.

The DV for calcium is 1,000 milligrams. But the amount that you need depends on your age, sex, and other factors. While men between the ages of 25 and 65, and women between the ages of 25 and 50, need 1,000 milligrams of calcium a day, men and women over 65 need 1,500 milligrams. Women who are postmenopausal and taking estrogen need 1,000 milligrams. Pregnant women or those who are breastfeeding need 1,200 to 1,500 milligrams a day.

## Help for Cancer

Fruits and vegetables have gotten the most glory as cancer-fighting foods, and rightly so. Still, drinking skim or low-fat milk may also play a protective role.

Researchers at Roswell Park Cancer Institute, led by Dr. Mettlin, asked 4,634 people with and without cancer how many glasses of whole milk, skim milk, or reduced-fat (2-percent) milk they drank a day. They found that those who drank skim or reduced-fat milk had lower risks of developing several types of cancers, including cancers of the stomach and rectum, then those who drank whole milk. "These reduced risks were most likely due to their consuming less dietary fat from milk as well as from other foods," says Dr. Mettlin.

Another study, sponsored by the American Cancer Society, found that women who drank skim or reduced-fat milk were three times less likely to develop ovarian cancer than women who drank more than a glass of whole milk a day.

Since a high intake of dietary fat is linked to cancer, it's not surprising that people who drank whole milk had the highest risks of cancer. What was surprising was that in both studies, people who didn't drink milk had higher risks of cancer than those who drank skim or reduced-fat milk. So there may be something in milk that helps protect against this disease, says Dr. Mettlin.

## Liquid Nutrition

We've been talking about milk's role in preventing disease. Yet even for healthy, day-to-day living, milk is a truly nutritious food. Apart from its high calcium content, 1 cup of milk also contains 100 international units (IU) of vitamin D, 25 percent of the DV. Just as your bones need calcium to stay strong, they also need vitamin D, which helps the calcium get absorbed.

In addition, 1 cup of skim milk supplies about 400 milligrams of potassium, approximately 12 percent of the DV. Potassium is a key mineral for protecting against high blood pressure, stroke, and heart trouble. Milk also contains 0.4 milligram of riboflavin, more than 23 percent of the DV.

# Getting the Most

**Buy it in cartons.** While those translucent plastic jugs are a convenient way to carry milk home from the store, they also admit light, which destroys riboflavin and vitamin A. In fact, milk stored for one day in a translucent plastic jug loses 90 percent of its vitamin A and 14 percent of its riboflavin. Further, the action of light can give milk an off-taste that many people find unpleasant. So you may want to buy the cartons instead.

**Give your taste buds time to adjust.** While some people take to skim milk right away, others loathe the taste, at least at first. To make skim milk part of your diet without shocking your taste buds, make the switch slowly. Try mixing a carton of whole milk with a carton of reduced-fat milk and drink that for a few weeks. Slowly reduce the amount of whole milk you add to the mix until you're drinking straight reduced-fat milk. When you're used to that, add skim milk to the reduced fat. Eventually, you'll be drinking—and enjoying—pure skim.

**Add some thickening.** One of the things people dislike about skim milk is its rather thin consistency. To make it thicker and creamier, try adding 2 to 4 tablespoons of nonfat milk powder into each cup of skim.

**Try a new brand.** If you're not happy with the milk you've been drinking, try one of the creamier versions. For example, Borden makes a product called Lite Line that's fat-free but tastes like reduced fat. Lite-Line is available in Texas and other selected regions. Or look for fat-free milk that's fortified with non-fat milk solids. It's labeled "protein fortified."

**Work it into your diet.** Even if milk isn't your favorite beverage, there are other ways to get it into your diet. For example, using skim milk instead of water when preparing oatmeal will boost your breakfast's calcium content from 20 to 320 milligrams.

# Mushrooms
## THE HEALING FUNGUS

When the rain falls, showering the earth with cool, clear water, it triggers the emergence of a miniature wonderland of woody, umbrella-shaped sprouts. Mushrooms, which are actually a fungus, literally crop up overnight, and are just as rapidly picked, both for their savory flavors and for their healing potential.

Mushrooms are so popular in Asian countries that they're sold by streetcart vendors, just as we sell corn dogs and Italian ice. But while Americans have been slow to embrace these meaty morsels, they're becoming increasingly commonplace, both in the kitchen and in research laboratories.

Scientists are discovering what natural healers have known for ages. Mushrooms, particularly the Asian varieties shiitake and maitake, not only are important sources of nutrients but also stimulate the immune system. Researchers say that they possibly can help fight cancer and high cholesterol, and perhaps even AIDS.

Unfortunately, the common white button mushroom, our favorite from the fungus family, has no known medicinal value. It does, however, supply good amounts of some key nutrients, like the B vitamins.

## A Cap on Cancer

Long esteemed in Japan for their reputed tumor-shrinking abilities, shiitake mushrooms have been attracting global attention because of the cancer-fighting compound that they contain.

These large, meaty black mushrooms contain a polysaccharide, or complex sugar, called lentinan. Polysaccharides are large molecules that are similar in structure to bacteria, explains Robert Murphy, R.N., a naturopathic doctor in private practice in Torrington, Connecticut. When you eat shiitake mushrooms, your immune system starts amassing an army of infection-fighting cells. "In essence, they fool the immune system into kicking into action," he says. Researchers have found that when they feed lentinan in the form of dried mushroom powder to laboratory animals with tumors, they can inhibit tumor growth by 67 percent.

Researchers are also looking at the maitake mushroom, also known as hen of the woods or the dancing mushroom. Like shiitakes, maitake mushrooms have a centuries-old reputation for being helpful in treating people with cancer. Only recently are they getting the attention that they deserve in Western nations.

The active polysaccharide in maitake mushrooms, called beta-glucan or D-fraction, has been highly effective in shrinking tumors in laboratory animals—maybe even more effective than lentinan, say experts.

The question that remains is, If they seem to be effective when taken as a powder, are they also effective when eaten whole? And do you have to eat a forestful to get the benefits?

"We don't know the precise benefit of eating them," says Dr. Murphy. "You definitely get some of these polysaccharides that activate the immune system when you eat a healthy serving—about a half-cup—of these mushrooms. Whenever I work with cancer patients, I use a concentrate of maitake D-fraction, and I tell people that they can go to the market and buy shiitake and maitake mushrooms and include them in their diets." Both types are usually found in Asian food stores and some supermarkets.

## IMMUNITY BOOSTING AND AIDS

Because the shiitake and maitake mushrooms have proven so effective in bolstering the immune system, some scientists have tested their mettle, with some success, against HIV, the virus that causes AIDS.

In laboratory studies, an extract of the maitake mushroom's beta-glucan was able to prevent HIV from killing T cells, the immune system's crucial white blood cells. "The bottom line is that eating these mushrooms on a regular basis seems to be a very good way to keep your immune system up and running," says Dr. Murphy.

## CUTTING CHOLESTEROL

If your cholesterol levels are hovering near the danger zone—200 and above—you might want to consider making mushrooms a regular side dish on your dinner table.

During the 1970s and 1980s, human and animal studies in Japan showed that one of the compounds in shiitake mushrooms, eritade-nine, could effectively lower cholesterol levels. More recently, re-searchers from Slovakia have found that by feeding mice 5 percent of their diets in dried mushrooms, particularly oyster mushrooms, they could reduce blood cholesterol by 45 percent, even when the mice were given high-cholesterol foods.

Researchers still can't say how many mushrooms people have to eat to get the same effect. But experts agree that adding a couple of these large, meaty morsels to your plate each day certainly can't hurt, and it may help play a role in bringing your cholesterol levels down.

## A BOOST OF Bs

Mushrooms offer two important B vitamins, niacin and riboflavin, that are not often found in vegetables. For once, the common white button mushroom may be a key player. While dried shiitake mush-rooms have a higher nutrient concentration, they also have a strong flavor; most people won't use them in large quantities. But white mush-rooms, with their mild taste, can be eaten with virtually every meal.

Niacin is important because it helps your body form the enzymes needed to convert sugars into energy, to use fats, and to keep your tis-sues healthy. It's generally found in whole grains and lean meats. But white button mushrooms are a good source, containing 4 milligrams of niacin, 20 percent of the Daily Value (DV).

Like niacin, riboflavin is a "helper nutrient." It's needed to convert other nutrients, like niacin, vitamin $B_6$, and folate, into usable forms. If you're low on riboflavin, you could also be low on these other nu-trients. A half-cup of sliced, boiled white mushrooms contains 0.2 milligram of riboflavin, 12 percent of the DV.

## Getting the Most

**Cook 'em up.** For both taste and nutrition, mushrooms are better cooked than raw. This is because they are mostly water. When you cook them, you remove the water and concentrate the nutrients as well as the flavor. Plus, cooking breaks down the mushrooms' cell walls so that the nutrients are more easily absorbed by your body.

**Eat the exotic.** To get optimal healing power from mushrooms, stick to Asian varieties, particularly shiitake and maitake, say experts. Other mushrooms that may provide therapeutic benefits are enoki, oyster, pine, and straw varieties.

# Nuts

## A SHELL GAME YOU CAN WIN

The ancient Persians believed that eating five almonds before drinking alcoholic beverages would prevent intoxication, or at least the hangover that might follow. They also believed that almonds would ward off witches and stimulate milk production in nursing mothers.

As nutty as this seems today, it's not surprising that ancient civilizations took their nuts seriously. Nuts are a compact source of energy and are easily stored through cold winters and hot summers, making them available throughout the year. They also contain a number of compounds that may help prevent heart disease and cancer.

### THE FAT FACTOR

Before we talk about the health benefits of nuts, it's important to discuss one of their potential drawbacks. While nuts are high in nutrients, they're also high in fat. One-third cup of nuts typically contains anywhere from 240 to 300 calories and 20 to 25 grams of fat.

Not all nuts are loaded with fat, but most are. The coconut, for example, contains a lot of fat, and most of it is the dangerous saturated kind. "On the other end of the spectrum is the chestnut, which is extremely low in fat and almost all of it is unsaturated," says Joan Sabaté, M.D., Dr. P.H., chairman of the department of nutrition and associate professor of nutrition and epidemiology at Loma Linda University School of Public Health in California.

"It's very unfortunate that people shun nuts just because they're high in calories," Dr. Sabaté adds. "The trick to eating nuts is not overdoing it—fitting them wisely into a healthy eating plan."

Even though nuts mainly contain a healthy form of fat, it's important not to eat too many of them. Or if you do, be sure to get less of other, less healthy fats, such as butter, hydrogenated margarines, and nutrient-empty snack foods such as chips and cookies, Dr. Sabaté says.

## GOOD FOR THE HEART

One great thing about nuts is that they contain a number of compounds that help keep the arteries open and blood flowing smoothly.

It was quite by accident that researchers at Loma Linda University discovered that eating nuts seems to protect against heart disease. They asked the 26,000 members of the Seventh-Day Adventist Church, an extremely health-conscious bunch, to indicate the frequency with which they ate 65 food items. As it turns out, the Adventists are very fond of nuts. Twenty-four percent ate nuts at least five times a week. In the population at large, only 5 percent of people eat them that often.

As the researchers discovered, this difference in nut consumption made a colossal difference in heart disease risk. Eating nuts just one to four times a week reduced the risk of dying from artery-clogging heart disease by 25 percent. People who ate them five or more times per week slashed their risks in half.

Researchers aren't sure which nuts made the most difference. Among the most popular choices were peanuts, almonds, and walnuts. (Even though peanuts are technically a legume, they're nutritionally similar to nuts and, in fact, are sometimes referred to as groundnuts.)

What is it about nuts, which are dripping with oil, that amazingly defats arteries? "With a few exceptions, most nuts are high in monounsaturated and polyunsaturated fats," says Dr. Sabaté. "When these types of fats replace saturated fats in the diet, they can help lower total cholesterol as well as the unhealthy low-density lipoprotein (LDL) cholesterol." At the same time, nuts don't affect levels of the heart-healthy high-density lipoprotein (HDL) cholesterol.

Another thing that makes nuts healthy for the heart is an amino acid called arginine. Some arginine may be converted in the body to nitric oxide, a compound that helps expand the blood vessels. In fact, it acts much like the drug nitroglycerin, which is used to rapidly dilate arteries to permit more blood to reach the heart. Nitric oxide also appears to help keep the platelets in blood from clumping, which can further reduce heart disease risk.

"Nuts are also high in vitamin E, which may keep LDL cholesterol from oxidizing," says Dr. Sabaté. This is the process that makes cholesterol more likely to stick to artery walls and block blood flow. Nuts have more vitamin E than any other food, with the exception of oils.

Almonds and walnuts are particularly good choices. One-third cup of either nut contains about 12 international units, or 40 percent of the Daily Value (DV).

Nuts also contain generous amounts of heart-healthy copper and magnesium. Magnesium appears to regulate cholesterol and blood pressure as well as heart rhythms, while copper may play a role in lowering cholesterol.

## PREVENTING CANCER

Just as nuts contain compounds that may help prevent heart disease, they also contain compounds that may help stop cancer.

Walnuts, for example, contain a compound called ellagic acid that appears to battle cancer on several fronts. "Ellagic acid is a good antioxidant, disabling harmful oxygen molecules, called free radicals, that are known to instigate the cancer process," says Gary D. Stoner, Ph.D., director of the cancer chemoprevention program at the Ohio State University Comprehensive Cancer Center in Columbus. Ellagic acid also helps detoxify potential cancer-causing substances, while at the same time helping to prevent cancer cells from dividing.

In one study, laboratory animals given ellagic acid as well as a cancer-causing substance were 33 percent less likely to develop esophageal cancer than animals given only carcinogens. In another study, laboratory animals were 70 percent less likely to develop liver tumors when they were given purified ellagic acid.

## A NUTRITIONAL PAYLOAD

All nuts are richly endowed with protein, and most contain a generous supply of vitamins and minerals as well as dietary fiber.

While the plain old peanut doesn't hit the charts for healing potential, it's the highest in protein of any nut, with $^1/_3$ cup containing more than 11 grams, 22 percent of the DV. That's more protein than you'll get from the same amount of beef or fish. Better yet, the protein in peanuts is a complete protein, meaning that it contains all the essential amino acids we can't do without. Brazil nuts, cashews, walnuts, and almonds also are good sources of protein, each containing at least 6 grams in $^1/_3$ cup, 12 percent of the DV.

In addition, all nuts are a good source of fiber, with $^1/_3$ cup typically containing 1 to 2 grams—about the amount in a similar-size serving of Cheerios. Among the most fiber-rich nuts are pistachios (nearly 5 grams per $^1/_3$ cup, almost 20 percent of the DV), and almonds (just over 6 grams, about 24 percent of the DV).

# Oats

## MOPPING UP CHOLESTEROL

You're hearing it straight from the horse's mouth: Oats are good food.

If it weren't for the horse, in fact, we probably wouldn't even know about oats, to say nothing of the great health benefits they provide. When horses were introduced in various parts of the world, oats went along as their feed. Not surprisingly, however, humans were a bit reluctant to take a taste. Samuel Johnson's 1755 *Dictionary of the English Language* defined oats as "a grain which in England is generally given to horses, but which in Scotland supports the people." It seems that the Scots were ahead of their time.

Oats are a very healthy grain. For one thing, unlike wheat, barley, and other grains, processed oats retain the bran and germ layers, which is where most of the nutrients reside. In addition, oats contain a variety of compounds that have been shown to reduce heart disease, fight cancer, lower blood sugar, improve insulin sensitivity, and help with dieting. And while the research is very preliminary, there's some evidence that oats may be effective in fighting HIV, the virus that causes AIDS.

### HELP FOR HIGH CHOLESTEROL

For years, we've been hearing that oatmeal and oat bran can help lower cholesterol, a critical move in reducing the risk of heart disease. Studies consistently show that getting more oats in the diet not only lowers total cholesterol but, more encouragingly, selectively lowers the bad low-density lipoprotein (LDL) cholesterol while leaving the beneficial high-density lipoprotein cholesterol alone.

Oats contain a type of soluble fiber called beta-glucan, which traps dietary cholesterol within a sticky gel in the intestine. Since this gel isn't absorbed by the body, it passes through the intestine, taking unwanted cholesterol with it.

Soluble fiber isn't the only thing doing the trapping. Oats also contain compounds called saponins, which in preliminary animal studies appear to bind to cholesterol and usher it out of the body. Saponins also glom onto bile acids. This is good because high levels of bile acids can cause cholesterol levels to rise.

"We used to think that saponins had only negative effects on the body," says Joanne L. Slavin, Ph.D., professor of nutrition at the University of Minnesota in St. Paul. "In fact, we call them antinutrients because they inhibit the absorption of various nutritional substances. But their positive health benefits are clearly stronger than their negative attributes."

It doesn't take a loaf of oats to lower cholesterol. Having about $^3/_4$ cup of dry oatmeal (which cooks up to about $1^1/_2$ cups) or just under $^1/_2$ cup of dry oat bran (which cooks up to about 1 cup) a day can help lower total cholesterol 5 percent. That means, for example, reducing a 250 cholesterol reading to 238, or a 300 reading to 285.

## A STABLE OF PROTECTION

Like all plant foods, oats contain a variety of compounds that provide different kinds of protection. Three of these compounds—tocotrienols (related to vitamin E), ferulic acid, and caffeic acid—are antioxidants. That is, they help control cell-damaging particles called free radicals, which, when left unchecked, can contribute to heart disease, cancer, and certain eye diseases.

Tocotrienols, which are richly abundant in oats, pack at least two punches against heart disease. They're very effective at stopping oxidation, the process that causes LDL cholesterol to turn rancid and stick to artery walls. Indeed, tocotrienols are 50 percent more powerful than vitamin E, says David J. A. Jenkins, M.D., Sc.D., Ph.D., professor of nutritional sciences and medicine at the University of Toronto. In addition, tocotrienols act on the liver, which might turn down the body's own production of cholesterol.

## BATTLING CANCER

Some of the same compounds in oats that protect against heart disease may also help prevent cancer, says A. Venket Rao, Ph.D., professor of nutrition at the University of Toronto.

We've already discussed how the saponins in oats bind to bile acids. This is important because, while bile acids are necessary for the absorption and digestion of fat, they also cause problems. In the large intestine, they get converted by bacteria into a form called secondary bile acids. Secondary bile acids can damage intestinal cells, possibly setting in motion the events that lead to cancer. "By binding up bile acids and reducing the amount that can be transformed into a toxic version, saponins may help lower cancer risk," says Dr. Rao.

In addition, saponins appear to strengthen the immune system, making the body better able to detect and deactivate foreign invaders such as bacteria, viruses, and cancer cells. "In animal experiments, the addition of saponins to the diet increased the number of natural killer cells, which translates into a stronger immune surveillance system," says Dr. Rao.

Other compounds in oats protect against cancer in much the same way that they help prevent heart disease—by neutralizing cell-damaging free radicals before they cause harm.

Finally, oats contain generous amounts of a compound called phytic acid, says Dr. Slavin. "Although we haven't identified the exact mechanism, there's some evidence that phytic acid binds up certain reactive minerals, which may be important in preventing colon cancer."

## KEEPING BLOOD SUGAR STEADY

Another benefit of oats is that they appear to help keep the body's blood sugar levels in balance. This is important for the estimated 21 million Americans with impaired glucose tolerance, a condition that is similar to diabetes and that increases the risks of heart disease and strokes.

In people with this condition, blood sugar levels are higher than they should be, but not so high that the people are actually diabetic. Yet even slightly elevated blood sugar levels may be cause for concern because they cause the body to pump out larger amounts of insulin to bring them down. The resulting condition, called *hyperinsulinemia*, increases the risk of developing artery-clogging heart disease.

The soluble fiber in oats lays down a protective gummy layer in the intestine. This slows the rate at which carbohydrates are absorbed by the body, which in turn helps keep blood sugar levels stable. In addition, soluble fiber appears to reduce the output of hormones in the digestive tract, which indirectly lowers the body's production of insulin.

Here's an additional benefit of the soluble fiber in oats. Because it soaks up lots of water, it creates a feeling of fullness. This means that when you eat oats, you feel satisfied longer and so are more likely to eat less, which is good news for anyone who's trying to lose weight.

## HELP FOR HIV

Although the evidence is still preliminary, the saponins in oats may be effective in disabling HIV, the virus that causes AIDS.

It's long been a puzzling fact that while some people infected with HIV develop AIDS relatively quickly, others don't become sick for years. Scientists are working to discover what makes HIV stronger, or more virulent, in some people.

It could be that various compounds found in food, including the saponins in oats, may play a role in squelching HIV. "Although this research is in its very early stages, it certainly is something to pursue," says Dr. Rao.

## Getting the Most

**Eat for convenience.** Unlike many foods, in which the processed versions are often the least nutritious, oats retain their goodness in different forms. So when time is an issue, go ahead and enjoy quick oats. They provide just as many vitamins and minerals as the traditional, slower-cooking kind. Keep in mind, however, that quick oats do contain more sodium than their slower-cooking kin.

**For protein, take your pick.** Both rolled oats and oat bran are good sources of protein. One cup of cooked oat bran contains 7 grams of protein, 14 percent of the Daily Value (DV), while a serving of rolled oats has 6 grams, 12 percent of the DV.

**Cut calories with bran.** When you're trying to eat lean, oat bran is often a better choice than oatmeal. A 1-cup serving of cooked oat bran contains 87 calories, whereas the same amount of oatmeal has 145.

# Olive Oil

## AN ELIXIR FOR YOUR HEART

Researchers were amazed more than 40 years ago when they first started studying Greeks living on the island of Crete. Even though the traditional Greek diet is very high in fat, people had exceptionally low rates of heart disease.

Since then, doctors have looked at every factor they can think of to see what would explain the Greeks' remarkably good health. One of the answers, it appears, is olive oil. "They have to be doing something right, and olive oil seems to play a critical role," suggest Dimitrios Trichopoulos, M.D., professor of epidemiology and cancer prevention at the Harvard School of Public Health.

We would do well to follow their example. Olive oil not only appears to lower the risk of heart disease, it may reduce the risk of breast cancer as well.

## A BETTER FAT

Olive oil is a monounsaturated fat. Doctors aren't sure why, but replacing saturated fats in the diet with olive oil lowers levels of low-density lipoprotein (LDL) cholesterol while leaving the beneficial high-density lipoprotein cholesterol alone.

The olive oil–loving Greeks eat very little butter or margarine, Dr. Trichopoulos adds. What's more, their main meals usually consist of vegetables or legumes instead of meats. So even though they use a lot of olive oil, they get very little saturated fat.

Here's the payoff. One scientific project, called the Seven Countries Study, found that while 46 percent of deaths among middle-aged American men were due to heart disease, the number in Crete was a mere 4 percent—more than 10 times lower.

## CHEMICALS FOR THE HEART

It's not only the monounsaturated fat that makes olive oil so good for the heart. It also contains other disease-fighting compounds that can stop damage in the arteries before it starts.

Here's why. The body naturally produces harmful oxygen molecules called free radicals. These molecules damage LDL cholesterol in the bloodstream, making it more likely to stick to artery walls. But several of the compounds in olive oil, such as polyphenols, are powerful antioxidants. This means that they're able to disable free radicals before they do damage, Dr. Trichopoulos explains. As a result, getting more olive oil in your diet can help keep your arteries clear.

## A WOMAN'S BEST FRIEND

Even though olive oil is best known for protecting the heart, evidence suggests that it may play a role in protecting the breasts as well. In a study of more than 2,300 women, researchers from the Harvard School of Public Health and the Athens School of Public Health in Greece found that women who used olive oil more than once a day had 25 percent lower risks of breast cancer compared to those who used it less often. And in fact, women in Greece are much less likely to die of breast cancer than their American counterparts.

"We're still not certain what accounts for this apparent protective effect," says Dr. Trichopoulos. Olive oil is rich in vitamin E, which has been shown to stop cellular damage that can lead to cancer. And of course, the same polyphenols that help prevent free radicals from damaging the heart may play a role in preventing cancer as well.

# Getting the Most

**Look for extra-virgin.** All olive oils are high in monounsaturated fats, but they don't contain equal amounts of disease-fighting polyphenols. To get the most of these compounds, look for olive oil labeled "extra-virgin." This type of oil is made from the first pressing of perfectly ripe olives, which leaves the polyphenols in and the bitter acids out.

**Keep it cold.** Because people don't always use a lot of olive oil, it tends to go bad on the shelf, giving up both its good taste and its protective compounds. To keep olive oil fresh, store it in the refrigerator or another dark, cool place. Bringing it to room temperature will quickly restore its pourable nature.

# Onion Family

## ROOTS OF GOOD HEALTH

Scene: The Civil War, 1864. The Union soldiers are ailing with dysentery. General Ulysses S. Grant wires a directive to the War Department to save his troops:

"I will not move my army without onions!"

Three trainloads are shipped the next day. The rest is history.

Sure, it's a stretch to say that onions won the war between the states. And scientists haven't proven that onions can stave off dysentery. But they do know that onions and their savory siblings—such as leeks, shallots, scallions, and other members of the allium family—contain dozens of compounds that could have helped protect the soldiers from a host of other serious conditions, including cancer, high blood pressure, heart disease, high cholesterol, and asthma.

So grab an onion, a sharp knife, and a hanky and start chopping your way to better health.

### ONION RINGS AND HEART STRINGS

Don't be offended the next time your honey suggests you "go Dutch" when you go out to dinner. He may be suggesting you take a cue from a group of heart-healthy men who ate their fill of onion-laden delights as part of a groundbreaking study in the Netherlands.

In this much-acclaimed study, researchers found that men who ate a quarter-cup of onions a day, along with an apple and four cups of tea, had one-third the risk of dying from heart attacks compared to those who ate the least amounts of these foods.

What's so important about onions? Wrapped beneath their papery skins are dozens of compounds that help lower cholesterol, thin the blood, and prevent hardening of the arteries—all of which can go a long way toward preventing heart disease.

The first family of heart-healthy compounds in onions is the flavonoids. Flavonoids are substances in plants that research has shown to have potent antioxidant powers, meaning that they help prevent disease by sweeping up harmful, cell-damaging oxygen molecules called free radicals, which naturally accumulate in your body.

One particular onion-dwelling flavonoid called quercetin has been shown to help knock out heart disease in two ways. One, it helps prevent the dangerous low-density lipoprotein form of cholesterol from oxidizing, which is the process that makes it stick to artery walls. Two, it helps prevent platelets in blood from sticking together and forming harmful clots.

A second group of protective compounds in onions are the same ones that make you cry—the sulfur compounds. Experts say that these compounds raise your levels of beneficial high-density lipoprotein cholesterol, which helps keep plaque from sticking to artery walls. At the same time, they lower levels of dangerous blood fats called triglycerides, which helps make blood thinner, keeping your blood pressure in the safety zone.

You don't need a lot of onions to keep your pump primed with protective compounds. In fact, studies show that you can reap the benefits by eating just one medium onion, raw or cooked, a day.

## CANCER PROTECTION

You can hold the pickles if you like, but when you're looking for cancer protection, don't skimp on the onions. They may be a key player in cancer prevention, especially cancers of the gastrointestinal tract, say experts.

"The primary flavonoid found in onions—quercetin—actually halts the progression of tumors in the colons of animals," says Michael J. Wargovich, Ph.D., professor of medicine at the M. D. Anderson Cancer Center at the University of Texas in Houston. This means that onions do double duty in suppressing tumors, because the sulfur compounds also fight cancer, adds Dr. Wargovich.

In a large study in the Netherlands, researchers looked at the diets of nearly 121,000 men and women. The more odoriferous bulbs these onion-loving Hollanders included in their daily diets, the lower their risks of stomach cancer.

Scientists suspect that onions prevent cancer not only by putting the brakes on tumor development but also by stomping out harmful bacteria that may get stomach cancer started.

# A Good Kind of Onion Breath

Putting a few layers of raw onions on your turkey burger can give you industrial-strength breath, but those very same onions also may give people with asthma or other respiratory ailments clearer airways.

"There are sulfur compounds in onions that inhibit the allergic, inflammatory response like that seen in asthma," says Eric Block, Ph.D., professor of chemistry at the State University of New York at Albany.

Although more research needs to be done on onions' asthma-attacking abilities, you can see the anti-inflammatory effect for yourself. The next time you have an insect bite or other type of minor inflammation on your skin, rub a cut onion on it. This should help reduce the inflammation, says Dr. Block.

You only need to eat a few servings of onions a day to keep your breathing passages free and clear. "Unlike some foods, where it's just not conceivable that you could eat enough to produce a significant effect, you can with onions," says Dr. Block. "If you like onions, you can consume them in pretty large quantities. And there's good evidence that you should."

# Combined Benefits

Whether you're eating for health or good taste, there's no reason to limit yourself to onions. Scallions, shallots, and other allium vegetables not only pack the same sulfur compounds and flavonoids as their bigger brothers, they also have a few of their own nutrients that can help fight disease and boost immunity.

Scallions, also called spring or green onions, are actually just young, underdeveloped onions. But they are higher in nutrients, particularly folate and vitamin C, than their adult counterparts.

A half-cup of chopped raw scallions provides 32 micrograms, or 8 percent of the Daily Value (DV) of folate, a nutrient that's essential for normal tissue growth and that may protect against cancer, heart disease, and birth defects. In that half-cup you'll also get more than 9 milligrams (almost 16 percent of the DV) of vitamin C, an immunity-boosting antioxidant nutrient that helps vacuum up tissue-damaging oxygen molecules in the body.

Shallots, another miniature member of the allium family, are similar to garlic cloves in that they come in a cluster of bulbs that are covered in brownish or reddish thick skin. Indeed, they taste like a combination of onions and garlic.

As with garlic, you probably won't want to eat large amounts of shallots in one sitting. And fortunately, you don't need to. Just 1 tablespoon of chopped shallots contains 600 international units of vitamin A, 12 percent of the DV. This essential nutrient helps keep immunity strong and also guards against vision problems associated with aging, like cataracts and night blindness.

# Getting the Most

**Add some color.** To get the most nutrients from your daily dose of onions, experts say, eat several different kinds. Red and yellow onions and shallots have the highest flavonoid content, while white onions have the least.

**Save your breath.** If the fear of having horrific halitosis is keeping you from enjoying the health benefits of onions, here's a freshening tip. Eat a sprig of fresh parsley. This will help neutralize the sulfur compounds before they turn into offending breath. A breath freshener made with parsley seed oil can also help.

**Keep your eyes peeled.** Even if you like onions, you may not love them enough to eat a half-cup or so a day. That's why scientists are trying to develop new onion strains with high concentrations of flavonoids like quercetin. Experts aren't sure when these new onions will be on the market, but keep your eyes open for special displays at your supermarket.

# Oranges

## THE SWEET TASTE OF CITRUS

The orange is nearly the perfect fruit. Not only is it high in vitamin C and fiber; it's also rich in natural sugars for quick energy. And because it comes ready-wrapped in its own protective skin, you can eat it anywhere, anytime.

Yet oranges are more than just a wholesome (and convenient) food. They also contain a quartet of compounds—limonin, limonene, limonin glucoside, and hesperidin—that show promise for blocking cancer. Plus, they contain compounds that may be able to stop heart disease even before it starts.

## HELP FOR THE HEART

Studies have shown that the vitamins and other compounds in oranges are surprisingly effective antioxidants. That is, they're able to block free radicals, corrosive oxygen molecules in the body that can damage cells, before they do harm. This is important because free radical damage can set the stage for clogging of the arteries, a key risk factor for heart disease and stroke.

Vitamin C has long been recognized as a powerful antioxidant. Yet there appear to be other compounds in oranges that are even more powerful.

"We measured the total antioxidant capacity of oranges and found that vitamin C only accounted for maybe 15 to 20 percent of the total activity," says Ronald L. Prior, scientific program officer at the Jean Mayer USDA Human Nutrition Research Center on Aging at Tufts University in Boston. "The other compounds in oranges turned out to be very strong antioxidants—anywhere from three to six times as potent as vitamin C."

In one study researchers gave rats an extract from the peel and pith of oranges. The extract, which contained the compound hesperidin, significantly raised the animals' levels of healthful high-density lipoprotein cholesterol, while at the same time lowering the dangerous low-density lipoprotein cholesterol. If hesperidin works the same way in human tests, oranges could be used to help temper high cholesterol, one of the main risk factors for heart disease.

Hesperidin may have other benefits as well. In laboratory studies, for example, Brazilian researchers found that hesperidin was able to help stop inflammation. And since it doesn't damage the delicate stomach lining the way aspirin can, it someday could be used to help relieve swelling in people who are sensitive to other anti-inflammatory drugs such as aspirin or ibuprofen.

## CANCER CONTROL

Laboratory studies have shown that the limonene found in oranges can help block certain cancers, says Bill Widmer, Ph.D., research scientist with the Florida Department of Citrus Research Center in Lake Alfred.

In a study at Duke University Medical Center in Durham, North Carolina, laboratory animals given a diet consisting of 10 percent limonene showed a 70 percent reduction in cancerous tumors. Among the tumors that remained, 20 percent shrank to less than half their former size.

In another study researchers at Cornell University in Ithaca, New York, fed animals with early stages of liver cancer an extract of orange juice concentrate from which the vitamin C had been removed. The incidence and size of precancerous lesions dropped 40 percent.

The research on limonene has been so promising that researchers in England are testing its effects on breast cancer.

"The way that limonene acts on tumor cells or lesions is really interesting and unique," says Michael Gould, Ph.D., professor of human oncology at the University of Wisconsin Medical School in Madison. Essentially, the compound gets cancer cells to self-destruct. It assists them in their own suicides.

## SEIZE THE Cs

Oranges are best known for their vitamin C, and with good reason. One orange contains about 70 milligrams of vitamin C, almost 117 percent of the Daily Value (DV). Vitamin C is critical not only for controlling harmful free radicals but also for aiding healing and boosting immunity. It's vitamin C's immune-boosting power that gives it its reputation for fighting the symptoms of a cold.

The vitamin also helps the body absorb iron from food, which is particularly important for women, who lose a little bit of iron (and blood) each month during menstruation.

In one large study, Gladys Block, Ph.D., professor of epidemiology and director of the public health nutrition program at the University of California, Berkeley, reviewed 46 smaller studies looking at the effects of vitamin C. Most of those studies found that people who got the most vitamin C had the lowest risks of cancer.

## FILLED WITH FIBER

An orange contains 3 grams of fiber, about 12 percent of the DV. Because insoluble fiber adds bulk to the stool, it can help relieve a host of intestinal problems, from constipation and hemorrhoids to diverticulosis. By speeding digestion, it can also help reduce the risk of colon cancer.

Oranges also contain a second form of fiber, called soluble fiber. This type of fiber, which includes pectin, breaks down to form a gel-like barrier in the small intestine. Studies show that it can help lower cholesterol as well as help control changes in blood sugar, critical for those with diabetes.

By eating more than seven oranges a day, you could lower your total cholesterol by about 20 percent. Of course, it's unlikely that anyone likes oranges that much. But by eating a variety of fruits and vegetables, including oranges whenever possible, you can do a lot to keep your cholesterol levels down.

# Getting the Most

**Stock your freezer.** Drinking orange juice is one of the easiest ways to get more vitamin C in your diet. Fresh juice is delicious, but it's also a bother to make. Fortunately, frozen juice retains most of the nutrients. In fact, since juice manufacturers squeeze every last drop from their fruit, a lot of the compounds in the peel wind up in the concentrate, providing additional health benefits along with good taste.

**Eat the sections.** Half of an orange's pectin is contained in the albedo, the inner white spongy layer that lies right under the colorful part of the skin. So don't be too neat when you eat. Eating a little of this spongy layer with each section will provide more of this important fiber.

# Parsnips
## UNSUNG HEROES

Parsnips might as well be called Pursed Lips for the reaction that these strong-tasting, oddly sweet vegetables often get. And they certainly won't win any awards for Best-Looking Vegetable in Show. They look like carrots that have seen a ghost.

But despite parsnips' strong flavor and pale appearance, their nutritional profile is quite attractive. A member of the parsley family, parsnips are good sources of folate, fiber, and phenolic acids, which have been shown in laboratory studies to help block cancer.

### FABULOUS FIBER

Whenever experts compile their "A" lists for healing substances, they invariably put dietary fiber near the top. And parsnips are an excellent source. One cup of cooked parsnips contains nearly 7 grams, 28 percent of the Daily Value (DV).

A little more than half of the fiber in parsnips is the soluble kind, which means that it becomes gel-like in the digestive system. This helps block the intestine from absorbing fats and cholesterol from foods. At the same time, it dilutes bile acids in the intestine, which can help prevent them from causing cancer. Parsnips also contain insoluble fiber, which speeds the rate at which stools move through the intestine. This is important because the less time bile acids are present in the intestine, the less likely they are to damage cells, causing changes that could lead to cancer.

The benefits of getting lots of fiber are well-known. In a review of more than 200 scientific studies, researchers found that getting more dietary fiber can protect against a wide variety of cancers, including cancer of the stomach, pancreas, and colon.

Fiber has shown similarly impressive ability to relieve or prevent many other conditions as well. Researchers have found that getting enough fiber in the diet can help prevent hemorrhoids and other intestinal conditions. Fiber can also curb the blood sugar swings that occur with diabetes.

## STROKE PREVENTION

Some nutrition experts say that too little folate is our number one nutritional deficiency, particularly among younger folks, who often eat large amounts of fast food that's largely devoid of vitamins. Parsnips are a good source of folate, with 1 cup containing 91 micrograms, 23 percent of the DV.

Getting enough folate has been shown to prevent certain birth defects. It's also strongly suspected of reducing the risk of stroke. Folate decreases blood levels of homocysteine, a chemical that may jam up the arteries and stop blood flow. Researchers at Harvard Medical School think that folate, along with the mineral potassium, played a key role in lowering the participants' risk of stroke in the landmark Framingham Heart Study.

The researchers found that men who ate the most produce had a 59 percent lower stroke rate than those who ate the least. Even those who ate just a little more produce reaped substantial benefits. The study found that folks who helped themselves to an extra three servings of fruits and vegetables a day lowered their risk of stroke by 22 percent.

Obviously, unless you truly have a passion for parsnips, it's unlikely that you'll ever eat three or more servings a day. But eating just a half-cup will provide not only fiber and folate but also 280 milligrams of potassium, 8 percent of the DV. This will go a long way toward keeping your arteries in the swim.

## THE ACID TEST

Scientists haven't uncovered the full wonders of parsnips yet, but preliminary research suggests that they may contain compounds that could have a direct impact on cancer cells in the body.

Along with carrots and celery, parsnips are members of the umbelliferae family. Foods in this family contain a number of natural compounds called phytonutrients, which have been shown in laboratory studies to block the spread of cancer cells. Chief among these are compounds called phenolic acids. What phenolic acids do is attach themselves to potential cancer-causing agents in the body, creating a bigger molecule—so big that the body can't absorb it.

Research has shown that members of the umbelliferae family can also fight cancer by inhibiting tumor growth.

The research is still preliminary, so it's not yet certain how effective parsnips are at blocking cancer. In the meantime, go ahead and enjoy parsnips for all the fiber and folate they contain.

# Getting the Most

**Trim the greens.** Before storing parsnips in the refrigerator, snip the greens from the top. Otherwise, the greens will draw moisture and nutrients from the root itself, according to Densie Webb, R.D., Ph.D., co-author of *Foods for Better Health*.

**Take a little more off the top and bottom.** Pesticides tend to accumulate around the tops and bottoms of parsnips, says Dr. Webb. Before cooking, it's a good idea to slice ¹/₄ to ¹/₂ inch off the top and bottom, she advises.

**Keep them cold.** Although some root vegetables keep well at room temperature, parsnips should be kept in the refrigerator or root cellar. "Keeping them cold and humid will keep them from drying out and losing some of their nutritional value," says Susan Thom, R.D., a resource spokesperson for the American Dietetic Association and a nutrition consultant in Brecksville, Ohio.

**Stock up ahead of time.** Parsnips will keep for a couple of weeks when stored in the refrigerator in a perforated or loosely closed plastic bag. "The longer you keep them in storage, the sweeter they get," says Thom. "That's because some of the starch turns to sugar. Unlike most vegetables, which deteriorate pretty quickly, they make a nice hardy vegetable to keep around."

**Boil before peeling.** Some of the nutrients in parsnips are water-soluble and are quickly lost during cooking. "They're fragile in boiling water—some of those vitamins float away," says Anne Dubner, a spokeswoman for the American Dietetic Association and a nutrition consultant in Houston.

In fact, you can lose almost half the water-soluble nutrients by cooking peeled parsnips. The solution, of course, is to cook them unpeeled. Once they're tender, let them cool, then scrape or peel the skin away.

# Pears

## THE CHOLESTEROL-
## FIGHTING FRUIT

When it comes to good health, you would think that pears would have more in common with apples and oranges than with a bowl of beans. But as it turns out, pears (along with beans) contain a type of dietary fiber that is very effective for lowering cholesterol.

Pears contain lignin, an insoluble fiber that helps usher unwanted cholesterol out of the body. Lignin acts like Velcro, trapping cholesterol molecules in the intestine before they get absorbed into the bloodstream. And because lignin can't pass through the intestinal wall, it goes into the stool, taking cholesterol along with it, explains Mary Ellen Camire, Ph.D., associate professor and chair of the department of food science and human nutrition at the University of Maine in Orono.

The insoluble fiber in pears serves another useful purpose. Insoluble fiber, as the name suggests, doesn't dissolve in the intestine. What it does, however, is absorb large amounts of water. This causes stools to pass more easily and quickly through the digestive tract, which helps prevent constipation and hemorrhoids and also reduces the risk of colon cancer.

Pears contain another type of fiber, called pectin, which is the same stuff you add to jellies and jams to help them jell. Pectin is a soluble fiber, meaning that it dissolves in the intestine, forming a sticky, gel-like coating. As with lignin, pectin binds to cholesterol in the intestine, causing it to be removed in the stool. This reduces the amount of cholesterol that gets into the bloodstream.

When you add up all the fiber in a single pear, you get about 4 grams, which is more than you'd get in a serving of Common Sense Oat Bran cereal or even a bran muffin. Eating just two pears will provide about 32 percent of the Daily Value for fiber.

## SAVING MINERALS

We don't usually think of pears as being "bone food," but they contain a mineral, boron, that appears to play a role in keeping bones strong.

Researchers have discovered that getting enough boron can help prevent the loss of calcium in postmenopausal women. This is important because these women have a high risk of osteoporosis, the bone-thinning disease that's caused by a gradual loss of minerals from the body.

What's good for the bones is also good for the brain. In tests of memory, perception, and attention, people low in boron did not perform as well as when they had higher amounts. And a study done by researchers at the U.S. Department of Agriculture found that reflexes and mental alertness improved when people were given additional boron.

It doesn't take a lot of boron to get the benefits. Just 3 milligrams a day has been shown to help prevent the loss of calcium and keep the mind strong. While it's unlikely that you would ever get all your boron from pears—one pear contains a little more than 0.3 milligram—having at least five servings a day of a variety of fruits and vegetables, including pears, will provide all the boron your body needs.

# Getting the Most

**Keep it clothed.** Most of a pear's fiber is in the peel. By eating pears with the skin on, you'll get the full complement of fiber, along with the cholesterol-lowering benefits, Dr. Camire says.

**Fresh is better.** While canned pears are convenient, they don't provide anywhere near the benefits of fresh, says Donald V. Schlimme, Ph.D., professor of nutrition and food science at the University of Maryland in College Park. For one thing, canned pears have been peeled, so they have lost most of their healing fiber. In addition, they may lose large amounts of nutrients during the canning process.

This isn't to say that you don't gain anything from canned pears. You do, although you probably don't want it. A serving of canned pears packed in heavy syrup delivers 25 percent more calories more than its fresh counterpart, Dr. Schlimme says.

# Peas

## SMALL WONDERS FOR HEALTH

Thanks to peas and an Austrian monk named Gregor Johann Mendel, we now have the science of genetics. Mendel found that when he bred two different peas together, their offspring had the features of both "parents." He concluded that physical characteristics could be passed down from generation to generation—not only in plants but in people as well.

Peas are more than an interesting scientific footnote, however. Researchers have found that they contain a powerful compound that can help prevent healthy cells from becoming cancerous. In addition, peas contain substances that can help lower cholesterol and ease symptoms of the common cold.

### IT'S HEALTHY BEING GREEN

The cancer-fighting compound in peas is called chlorophyllin, which is the pigment responsible for giving them their shiny green hue. Chlorophyllin (which is related to chlorophyll, the substance that allows plants to convert sunlight into food) has a special molecular shape that allows it to grab cancer-causing chemicals in the body. "When you eat peas, the chlorophyllin attaches to carcinogens and helps prevent them from being absorbed," says Mary Ellen Camire, Ph.D., associate professor and chair of the department of food science and human nutrition at the University of Maine in Orono.

Researchers haven't pinned down exactly how many peas you'd have to eat to get the most benefits from chlorophyllin, Dr. Camire says. You can't go wrong, however, by including them on your menu as often as possible, along with other bright, green vegetables. After all, the greener a vegetable is, the more chlorophyllin it contains.

## Helping Your Heart

Doctors have known for a long time that getting more dietary fiber is one of the best ways to lower cholesterol, and with it the risk for heart disease and other serious health problems. Green peas are an excellent source of fiber, with more than 4 grams in each half-cup serving.

Inside the intestine, the fiber in peas binds with bile, a digestive fluid produced by the liver, and traps it inside the stool. Since bile is very high in cholesterol, removing it from the body will automatically help bring cholesterol levels down.

Research suggests that eating peas can also bring down levels of triglycerides, blood fats that play a role in heart disease. A study in Denmark found that when people were given small amounts of pea fiber in addition to their usual diets, total tryglyceride levels fell almost 13 percent within two weeks.

## Pods of Good Health

Peas have always been a favorite in school cafeterias—not because they're fun to flip off a fork but because they contain an abundance of disease-fighting vitamins. A half-cup of green peas, for example, contains more than 11 milligrams of vitamin C, almost 19 percent of the Daily Value.

This is important because getting enough vitamin C in the diet has been shown to reduce the risk of cancer and heart disease. And when you have a cold, getting extra vitamin C will make the symptoms just a little more bearable.

# Getting the Most

**Fresh is finer.** Peas shucked right out of the pod have more vitamin C than those that come in a can because canned peas lose many of their nutrients during processing, says Donald V. Schlimme, Ph.D., professor of nutrition and food science at the University of Maryland in College Park.

**Visit the freezer case.** Fresh peas can be hard to come by at certain times of the year, but frozen peas are always available. While they lack some of the crispness of fresh, they're just as good for you because freezing keeps most of the nutrients, especially vitamin C, intact.

**Shuck the pods.** Even though edible-podded peas (such as sugar snap peas) contain large amounts of vitamin C, the peas themselves contain most of the fiber, folate, niacin, phosphorus, riboflavin, thiamin, and vitamin A. To get the most nutritional bang for your buck, it's better to eat a half-cup of peas than an equal serving of peas in the pod, Dr. Camire says.

**Turn on the steamer.** Whether you're using fresh or frozen peas, it's best to heat them by steaming rather than boiling. Boiling leaches nutrients out of peas into the cooking water. In addition, the high heat used in boiling may destroy some of the nutrients, particularly the vitamin C. If you don't have a steamer, heating them quickly in the microwave is a good alternative.

# Pineapple

## A TROPICAL CHAMP

When King Louis XIV of France was first presented with a pineapple—the most exotic and sought-after fruit in seventeenth-century Europe—he immediately took a huge bite. Unfortunately, His Greediness hadn't given his servants a chance to peel it, so he cut his royal lips on the prickly rind. This episode put an end to the royal cultivation of pineapple in France until Louis XV took the throne in 1715.

The pineapple-punctured potentate didn't know what he was missing. Stripping a pineapple of its spiny hide (or at least opening a can of the stuff) is well worth your time. Not only is pineapple a rich source of vitamin C, it also contains substances that keep bones strong and promote digestion.

### A JUICY BONE-BUILDER

You know that you need calcium to prevent osteoporosis, the bone-thinning disease that primarily affects postmenopausal women. What you may not know is that your bones need manganese as well.

The body uses manganese to make collagen, a tough, fibrous protein that helps build connective tissues like bone, skin, and cartilage. Research has shown that people deficient in manganese develop bone problems similar to osteoporosis. One study found that women with osteoporosis had lower levels of manganese than women who did not have the disease.

"Eating fresh pineapple or drinking pineapple juice is a good way to add manganese to your diet," says Jeanne Freeland-Graves, Ph.D., professor of nutrition at the University of Texas in Austin. A cup of fresh pineapple chunks or pineapple juice will give you over 2 milligrams of manganese, more than 100 percent of the Daily Value (DV).

## SWEETEN YOUR DIGESTION

Pineapple has a centuries-old reputation for relieving indigestion, and there may be good reasons for that. Fresh pineapple contains bromelain, an enzyme that helps digestion by breaking down protein. This might be important for some older people who have low levels of stomach acid, which is needed for protein digestion.

Even if you love pineapple, of course, it's unlikely you'd eat it after every meal. But if you are older and have frequent indigestion, adding a few pineapple slices to your dessert plate might help keep your stomach calm, says Joanne Curran-Celentano, R.D., Ph.D., associate professor of nutritional sciences at the University of New Hampshire in Durham.

## A GREAT SOURCE OF VITAMIN C

Few nutrients get as much attention as vitamin C, and for good reason. This vitamin is a powerful antioxidant, meaning that it helps thwart free radicals, unstable oxygen molecules that damage cells and contribute to the development of cancer and heart disease. In addition, the body uses vitamin C to make collagen, the "glue" that holds tissue and bone together. And when you have a cold, the first thing you probably reach for is vitamin C. It reduces levels of a chemical called histamine, which causes such cold symptoms as watery eyes and runny noses.

While pineapples aren't as rich in vitamin C as oranges or grapefruits, they're still excellent sources. One cup of pineapple chunks, for example, contains about 24 milligrams of vitamin C, 40 percent of the DV. Juice is even better. A glass of canned pineapple juice contains 60 milligrams, 100 percent of the DV.

# Getting the Most

**Buy it fresh.** Canned pineapple is convenient, but when you're eating it to soothe an upset stomach, the fresh fruit is best because the intense heat used in canning destroys the bromelain, says Dr. Taussig.

**Try a new variety.** The next time you're at the store, look for a "Gold" pineapple. Imported from Costa Rica, this variety is exceptionally sweet, and it has more than four times the vitamin C found in other varieties.

# Potatoes

## OUR SUPER STAPLE

Early in the history of the New World, in the Andes mountains of Peru and Bolivia, the people had a thousand names for the potato. It was that important.

In the 4,000 or so years since, the starchy tuber's reputation has peaked and dipped. The Spanish conquistadors thought the new root captivating enough to take back to the Old World. Within a few years, potatoes became standard fare on Spanish ships because they prevented scurvy. Once the potato arrived in Europe, though, its fortunes sagged, not because of any shortcomings of its own but because of its kinship with the deadly nightshade family, plants that had the reputation for being toxic. Potatoes were feared rather than appreciated.

Eventually, though, botanists and diners learned the whole story. Potatoes aren't remotely dangerous. Plus, they're a super food staple, making them the world's number one vegetable crop. In fact, it's not uncommon for people to eat potatoes, cooked in a variety of ways, with every meal.

"The potato has a little bit of almost everything," says Mark Kestin, Ph.D., chairman of the nutrition program at Bastyr University and affiliate assistant professor of epidemiology at the University of Washington, both in Seattle. "You could get many of your nutritional needs met from potatoes, if you had to," he adds.

## PEEL POWER

A potato's healing abilities start in the peel, which contains an anticarcinogenic compound called chlorogenic acid, says Mary Ellen Camire, Ph.D., associate professor and chair of the department of food science and human nutrition at the University of Maine in Orono. In laboratory studies, this particular acid has been shown to help the fiber in potatoes absorb benzo(a)pyrene, a potential carcinogen found in smoked foods such as grilled hamburgers.

"The acid in the food reacts with the carcinogen by basically binding it up and making too big a molecule for the body to absorb," Dr. Camire explains. "In our laboratory study, it prevented the carcinogen from being absorbed almost completely."

## SLASHING THE PRESSURE

We don't normally think of potatoes as being high in potassium, but in fact, a baked 7-ounce spud contains more than twice the potassium of one medium-size banana. One baked potato with the skin will give you about 1,137 milligrams of potassium, almost a third of the Daily Value (DV).

Potassium is important because it seems to calm the spiking effect that salt has on blood pressure. For some people, increasing potassium in their diets by eating potatoes could reduce the need for blood pressure medication, notes pharmacist Earl Mindell, R.Ph., Ph.D., professor of nutrition at Pacific Western University in Los Angeles and author of *Earl Mindell's Food as Medicine*. In one study of 54 people with high blood pressures, half added potassium-rich foods like potatoes to their diets, while the other half continued to eat their normal fare. By the end of the study, Dr. Mindell says, 81 percent of the potato-eaters were able to control their blood pressures with less than half the medication they had used previously.

## BLOOD SUGAR SAVIOR

We don't think of vitamin C as affecting our blood sugar, but there's emerging evidence that this powerful antioxidant vitamin, well-known for helping prevent heart disease, may be of help to people with diabetes. On top of this, vitamin C may also be effective in diminishing the damage to proteins caused by free radicals, dangerous oxygen molecules that damage tissues in the body.

In one study, researchers in the Netherlands found that men eating healthy diets, which were high not only in potatoes but also in fish, vegetables, and legumes, appeared to have lower risks for diabetes. It's not yet clear what the protective mechanism is, but researchers speculate that antioxidants, including vitamin C, may play a role in keeping excess sugar out of the bloodstream. One 7-ounce potato contains about 27 milligrams of vitamin C, about 45 percent of the DV.

Because potatoes are high in complex carbohydrates, they're also good for people who already have diabetes. Complex carbohydrates must be broken down into simple sugars before they're absorbed into the bloodstream. This means that the sugars enter the bloodstream in a leisurely fashion rather than pouring in all at once. This, in turn, helps keep blood sugar levels stable, which is a critical part of controlling the disease.

Further, potatoes can be key players in helping people with diabetes keep their weight down, an important benefit since being overweight makes it more difficult for the body to produce enough insulin, the hormone that helps transport sugars out of the bloodstream and into individual cells. At the same time, being overweight makes the insulin that the body does produce work less efficiently. What potatoes do is keep you full so that you're less likely to be hungry later on.

In a study of 41 hungry students at the University of Sydney in Australia, researchers found that spuds filled them up more than other foods, while at the same time delivering fewer calories. On a satiety scale that measured white bread at 100, oatmeal at 209, and fish at 225, potatoes were way ahead at 323.

# Getting the Most

**Keep the peel.** To take advantage of potatoes' cancer-fighting abilities, you really have to eat the peel, says Dr. Camire. This can be particularly important when eating grilled foods, which leave small amounts of cancer-causing substances on the food. It would be nice if you could get a fast-food burger on a potato-peel bun, says Dr. Camire. "That would help absorb the carcinogens from the grilling," she says.

A more practical solution is simply to add a baked potato or potato salad (with the peel) to your plate whenever you eat a grilled hamburger, a hot dog, or other smoky foods.

**Cook them carefully.** Although boiling is one of the most popular cooking methods for potatoes, it's perhaps the worst choice for preserving nutrients, since vitamin C and some B vitamins are pulled out of the potatoes and into the cooking water. In fact, boiling potatoes can result in losing about half the vitamin C, a quarter of the folate, and 40 percent of the potassium, says Marilyn A. Swanson, R.D., Ph.D., professor and head of the department of nutrition and food science at South Dakota State University in Brookings.

If you do boil potatoes, you can recapture some of the nutrients by saving the cooking water and adding it to other foods such as soups and stews.

Baking and steaming do a good job of tenderizing potatoes while at the same time preserving more of their nutrients. "Microwaving is your first choice," says Susan Thom, R.D., resource spokesperson for the American Dietetic Association and a nutrition consultant in Brecksville, Ohio.

**Prepare them late.** Busy cooks have traditionally peeled and sliced potatoes ahead of time, then submerged them in water to keep them from darkening. This may keep potatoes looking fresh, but it also strips valuable nutrients. "You lose some of the soluble vitamins in the water," says Mona Sutnick, R.D., a nutrition consultant in Philadelphia and a spokesperson for the American Dietetic Association.

# Prunes

## WORTH A SECOND LOOK

Prunes have an image problem. After all, these wrinkled, purple fruits are best known as a home remedy for constipation—not exactly a sexy angle for a snazzy marketing campaign. In fact, in an effort to burnish the prune's reputation, members of the prune industry have begun to call them dried plums.

It's unfortunate that the prune's dowdy image has prevented it from being more widely enjoyed. It may not be the most glamorous fruit on the market, but it's certainly one of the healthiest.

### NATURE'S LAXATIVE

Pharmacies stock dozens of medications for preventing and relieving constipation. But most of the time they really aren't necessary if you get in the habit of adding prunes to your daily diet. Prunes contain not just one but three different ingredients that work together to help keep your digestive system on track.

For starters, prunes are high in insoluble fiber, which is perhaps the key to preventing constipation. Since insoluble fiber isn't absorbed by your body, it stays in the digestive tract. And because it's incredibly absorbent, it soaks up large amounts of water, making stools larger and easier to pass. (Prunes also contain soluble fiber, the type that helps lower cholesterol and the risk of heart disease.) Just five prunes contain almost 3 grams of fiber, about 12 percent of the Daily Value (DV).

In addition, prunes contain a natural sugar called sorbitol. Like fiber, sorbitol soaks up water wherever it can find it, says Mary Ellen Camire, Ph.D., associate professor and chair of the department of food science and human nutrition at the University of Maine in Orono. Most fruits contain small amounts (usually less than 1 percent) of sorbitol. Prunes, however, are about 15 percent sorbitol, which explains why they're such a potent bulking agent and are often recommended for relieving constipation.

Finally, prunes contain a compound called dihydroxyphenyl isatin, which stimulates the intestine, causing it to contract. This process is essential for having regular bowel movements.

You don't need a lot of prunes to get the benefits. One daily serving—about five prunes—is all most people need to help themselves stay regular.

## ALL-AROUND PROTECTION

As with most fruits, prunes contain generous amounts of a variety of vitamins, minerals, and other healthful compounds.

One of the most healthful compounds in prunes is beta-carotene. Like vitamins C and E, beta-carotene is an antioxidant, meaning that it helps neutralize harmful oxygen molecules in the body. This is important because these molecules, known as free radicals, can eventually damage healthy cells throughout your body, possibly causing such serious health threats as heart disease and cancer. A serving of prunes contains almost 0.5 milligram of beta-carotene, about 3 percent of the recommended daily amount.

Prunes also contain generous amounts of potassium, a mineral that's essential for keeping blood pressure down. Studies have shown that when potassium levels decline, even for short periods of time, blood pressure rises. This is a dangerous situation because high blood pressure has been linked to conditions ranging from heart disease to stroke. Prunes are a very good source of potassium, with five prunes containing 313 milligrams, about 9 percent of the DV.

# Getting the Most

**For vitamins, drink the juice.** Although prune juice has less fiber than the whole fruit, it's a more concentrated source of vitamins. For example, five whole prunes contain more than 1 milligram of vitamin C, while a 6-ounce glass of juice contains almost 8 milligrams.

**For regularity, eat the fruit.** Since fiber is such an important part of digestive health, doctors recommend eating whole prunes, either fresh or canned, when you're trying to stay regular. While prune juice has also been used to help relieve constipation, it's somewhat less effective than the whole fruit.

# Pumpkin
## THE BETA-CAROTENE KING

*We have pumpkin at morning and pumpkin at noon.*
*If it were not for pumpkin, we should be undoon.*

This is a poem that the early American colonists chanted whenever they were overcome with appreciation for this oversize orange squash. Pumpkin was a popular food back then, and the early settlers ate a peck of it in pumpkin soup, pumpkin pie, and even pumpkin beer.

It's a different story now. We usually buy pumpkin as a Halloween decoration and then throw away the meat. If we actually eat pumpkin at all, it's mainly in Thanksgiving and Christmas pies.

That's a darn shame, since pumpkin is more than just a giant winter squash and a whittler's delight. It's also filled with powerful carotenoids like beta-carotene, which can help stop cellular damage before it leads to disease.

### GOOD FOR THE EYES—AND MORE

It's not just due to its size that pumpkin is called the king of squash. A half-cup of canned pumpkin has more than 16 milligrams of beta-carotene, 160 to 260 percent of the daily amount recommended by most experts. Pumpkin is also a source of lesser-known carotenoids such as lutein and zeaxanthin.

Carotenoids, which create the brilliant orange color of pumpkin, help protect the body by neutralizing harmful oxygen molecules known as free radicals. "Lutein and zeaxanthin are very potent free radical scavengers," says Paul Lachance, Ph.D., professor of nutrition and chairman of the department of food science at Rutgers University in New Brunswick, New Jersey. A diet high in antioxidants can help prevent many of the diseases associated with aging, including heart disease and cancer.

Lutein and zeaxanthin aren't found only in foods like pumpkin; they are also found in the lenses of the eyes. Studies suggest that eating foods high in these compounds may help block the formation of cataracts.

In one study, scientists at the Massachusetts Eye and Ear Infirmary in Boston compared the diets of elderly people who had advanced macular degeneration, a condition that leads to blurred vision, to the diets of those without the disease. The researchers found that those who ate the most carotenoid-rich foods had a 43 percent lower risk of getting this condition than folks who ate the least. Among people who already had macular degeneration, those who got the most carotenoids in their diets were less likely to develop a more serious form of the disease.

The beta-carotene in pumpkin helps protect the plant itself from diseases, from getting too much sunlight, and from other naturally occurring stresses. There's strong evidence that beta-carotene can help protect people from a variety of conditions as well. Research has shown, for example, that getting more beta-carotene in the diet can help protect against a variety of cancers, including cancers of the stomach, esophagus, lungs, and colon. This protective effect is enhanced by phenolic acids, which are chemicals in pumpkin that bind to potential carcinogens and help prevent them from being absorbed.

The beta-carotene in pumpkin may play a role in preventing heart disease as well. Some research suggests that people with diets high in fruits and vegetables that contain beta-carotene have a lower risk of heart disease than those whose diets supplied less.

For people prone to allergies or infections, eating regular helpings of pumpkin can help in yet another way, since the beta-carotene in pumpkin converts to vitamin A in the body. According to Susan M. Lark, M.D., in her book *Foods and Recipes for Women's Health*, vitamin A helps strengthen the immune system, which protects against developing respiratory disease and also helps prevent allergy attacks.

## THE WHOLE PICTURE

In addition to its rich stores of beta-carotene and other phytonutrients, pumpkin contains generous amounts of fiber. For example, while 1 cup of cornflakes contains 1 gram of fiber, a half-cup of canned pumpkin contains more than 3 grams, 6 percent of the Daily Value.

Iron is another pumpkin mainstay. A half-cup of pumpkin provides almost 2 milligrams of iron, about 20 percent of the Recommended Dietary Allowance (RDA) for men and 13 percent of the RDA for women. This is particularly important for women, who need to replenish their iron regularly due to menstruation.

Even richer in iron than the flesh are the pumpkin's seeds. One ounce—which consists of about 140 seeds, a huge handful—contains about 4 milligrams of iron, about 40 percent of the RDA for men and 27 percent of the RDA for women. What's more, that ounce of seeds has as much protein—9 grams—as an ounce of meat, says Susan Thom, R.D., a resource spokesperson for the American Dietetic Association and a nutrition consultant in Brecksville, Ohio.

Of course, you don't want to eat too many pumpkin seeds, since about 73 percent of the calories (there are 148 calories in an ounce of seeds) come from fat. But when you have a taste for a crunchy, highly nutritious snack, pumpkin seeds, in moderation, are a good choice.

# Getting the Most

**Consider it canned.** There's something about preparing a huge pumpkin that daunts even dedicated cooks and prevents them from utilizing its healing powers. An easy, convenient alternative is to buy canned pumpkin. Nutritionally, "it's almost equal to fresh," says Pamela Savage-Marr, R.D., spokesperson for the American Dietetic Association and a health education specialist at Oakwood Healthcare System in Dearborn, Michigan.

**Buy it tender.** When you have a taste for fresh pumpkin, be sure to shop for milder varieties, like the mini-sized Jack Be Littles. While large pumpkins are great for carving, they also tend to be tough and stringy, and most people don't enjoy them as much.

**Temper the taste.** Pumpkin is among the stronger-flavored squashes, and even people who like the taste can be overwhelmed by its potent presence. To get the most pumpkin into your diet, you may want to mellow the taste. One way to do this is to add about a tablespoon of orange juice or any other citrus juice during cooking, suggests Anne Dubner, R.D., a spokeswoman for the American Dietetic Association and a nutrition consultant in Houston.

**Love your leftovers.** There's no reason to force yourself to eat an entire pumpkin at one sitting—as though you could! Properly frozen, pumpkin retains virtually all its goodness and nutrition.

# Raisins

## A Handful of Health

Raisins may not be much to look at, but they do have an illustrious history. Prehistoric cave dwellers attributed religious powers to raisins. They made raisin necklaces and decorations and drew pictures of raisins on cave walls. As early as 1000 B.C., the Israelites used them to pay taxes to King David. Just try that with the IRS!

Raisins occupy a much humbler place in society today. But they're just as useful as ever. Backpackers and hikers appreciate raisins for being a high-energy, low-fat, very convenient snack. Raisins fit easily in a lunch box, and they don't get as mushy as bananas if you accidentally leave them in your desk drawer. And they almost never go bad, even when they're in the pantry for months at a time.

Raisins offer more than just convenience. Studies suggest that they can help lower blood pressure and cholesterol and even play a role in keeping digestion and blood healthy.

### LOWERING THE PRESSURE

If you have high blood pressure—or even if you don't, but you want to make sure your pressure stays in a healthy range—raisins are one of the best snacks you can buy. They're a good source of potassium, a mineral that has been shown to lower high blood pressure.

In one study researchers at Johns Hopkins Medical Institutions in Baltimore gave 87 African-American men either potassium supplements or blank pills. Those given the potassium saw their systolic pressure (the higher number) drop almost 7 points, while their diastolic pressure went down almost 3 points. While the amount of potassium given in the study was quite high—you'd have to eat about 3 cups of raisins to get the same amount—smaller amounts are also beneficial. Just $1/4$ cup of raisins contains 272 milligrams of potassium, almost 8 percent of the Daily Value (DV).

## IRON AND MORE

When we think of iron-rich foods, things such as red meat and liver usually come to mind. But raisins may be a better source, particularly for people who eat little or no meat. "If someone would ask me what food other than red meat I recommend for high iron, I would say raisins," says Donald V. Schlimme, Ph.D., professor of nutrition and food science at the University of Maryland in College Park.

Iron is essential for creating hemoglobin in red blood cells, which the body uses to transport oxygen. Although iron is readily available in food, women who are menstruating or pregnant often need extra amounts. A quarter-cup of raisins has 0.8 milligram of iron, more than 8 percent of the Recommended Dietary Allowance (RDA) for men and 5 percent of the RDA for women.

Like other dried fruits, raisins are also a good source of dietary fiber, with nearly 2 grams in 1/4 cup, about 8 percent of the DV. Not only does fiber help prevent everyday problems such as constipation and hemorrhoids; it also lowers cholesterol and the risk of heart disease.

In one study, researchers at the Health Research and Studies Center in Los Altos, California, asked people with high cholesterol to eat 3 ounces of raisins (a little more than a half-cup) a day as part of a high-fiber, low-fat diet. After a month, their total cholesterol dropped an average of more than 8 percent, while the harmful low-density lipoprotein cholesterol dropped 15 percent.

# Getting the Most

**Have a raisin combo.** Raisins contain a type of iron called non-heme iron, which is harder for the body to absorb than the heme iron found in meats. Eating raisins along with foods high in vitamin C, however, helps improve the absorption of nonheme iron. So the next time you're ready for a snack, have a piece of fruit or a glass of fruit juice along with the raisins. Or sprinkle them in a salad made with fruit or leafy greens.

**Shop for convenience.** To get the most raisins in your diet, nutritionists often recommend buying the snack-size packs. Due to their small size and the fact that raisins almost never go bad, they're perfect for tossing in your purse, glove compartment, or desk drawer.

# Rice

## A UNIVERSAL GRAIN

If there were just one food in every cook's pantry, it would probably be rice. Rice is the main ingredient in cuisines around the globe, with an estimated 40,000 varieties available worldwide. In the United States you can buy basmati rice from India and Pakistan, arborio rice from Italy, Valencia rice from Spain, and "sticky" rice from Japan. (Wild rice, incidentally, is really a grass, not a rice at all.)

The most nutritious kind of rice is brown rice, which contains abundant amounts of fiber, complex carbohydrates, and essential B vitamins, says Maren Hegsted, Ph.D., professor of human nutrition and food at Louisiana State University in Baton Rouge. Plus, it contains a powerful compound that helps reduce the amount of cholesterol produced by the body. Since high cholesterol is one of the biggest risk factors for heart disease, brown rice can play a key role in any heart-protection plan.

### STRIKE AT THE SOURCE

We often forget that the body actually needs small amounts of cholesterol for functions such as making cell walls, for example, and for manufacturing essential hormones. To supply the necessary amounts, the liver produces cholesterol every day. But when we eat a high-fat diet, the body churns out more cholesterol than it can use, and that's when the risk of heart disease goes up.

Getting more brown rice, Dr. Hegsted says, can help keep this from happening. The outer layer of brown rice, called the bran, contains a compound called oryzanol that has been shown to reduce the body's production of cholesterol. In fact, this compound is chemically similar to cholesterol-lowering medications.

In a study at Louisiana State University, people ate 100 grams (about 3¹/₂ ounces) of rice bran a day for three weeks. At the end of the study, researchers found that their cholesterol levels had dropped an average of 7 percent. Better yet, levels of harmful low-density lipoprotein cholesterol went down 10 percent, while levels of beneficial high-density lipoprotein cholesterol stayed relatively high.

A 10 percent drop in cholesterol may not sound like much, but doctors estimate that for every 1 percent you lower your cholesterol, your risk of heart disease drops 2 percent. This means that the rice-eaters lowered their risk of heart disease by 20 percent in only three weeks. "In combination with a low-fat diet, brown rice is one of the best foods you can eat for lowering cholesterol," says Dr. Hegsted.

## A Digestive Sponge

Brown rice is darker and more chewy than its light-colored cousin because it's wrapped in a nutritious outer skin—the part of the grain that's highest in fiber, says Christine Negm, R.D., nutritionist and director of technical services for Lundberg Family Farms, which produces rice in Richvale, California. A half-cup of brown rice contains about 2 grams of fiber, she says.

The fiber in brown rice is the insoluble kind that acts like a sponge in the intestine, soaking up large amounts of water, says Dr. Hegsted. This causes stools to get larger and wetter, so they pass more easily. Larger stools also move more quickly through the colon. This means that any harmful substances that they contain have less time to damage cells in the colon wall, which can reduce the risk of cancer. Researchers estimate that if people would increase the amount of fiber in their diets to 39 grams a day, colon cancer risk could drop 31 percent.

What's good for the colon is also good for the breasts. Since the fiber in brown rice binds with estrogen in the digestive tract, there's less of the hormone circulating in the bloodstream. This is important because high levels of estrogen have been shown to trigger changes in cells that can lead to breast cancer. A study by Australian and Canadian researchers found that women who ate 28 grams of fiber a day had a 38 percent lower risk of developing breast cancer than those getting half that amount.

## Giving Nature a Hand

The problem with white rice is that the nutritious outer layers are stripped away during processing, leaving behind a tender but less healthful grain. To bring it up to speed, manufacturers do a nutritional sleight of hand. They replace some of the nutrients, like niacin and thiamin, that the processing took out. As a result, white rice may contain more of these nutrients than nature put in.

A half-cup of white rice has 0.2 milligram of thiamin, a B vitamin that's essential for converting food into energy, and 2 milligrams of niacin, which aids in metabolism. Brown rice, by contrast, has only 0.1 milligram of thiamin and 1 milligram of niacin. "White rice is fortified to the max," Negm says.

What white rice is lacking, however, is the fiber. A half-cup serving contains a scanty 0.2 gram of fiber, 10 times less than an equal amount of brown rice. So when you're trying to get the most nutritional bang for your buck, brown rice is usually a better choice.

# Getting the Most

**Keep it cool.** Since brown rice is filled with oils, it quickly turns rancid when stored at normal room temperature, Dr. Hegsted says. To preserve the healing compounds, be sure to store brown rice in an airtight container in the refrigerator, where it will stay fresh for up to a year.

**Save the water.** Many of the important nutrients in brown and white rice leach into the water during cooking. To get these nutrients on your plate instead of pouring them down the drain, let rice cook until all the water is absorbed.

**Use it "dry."** Since the niacin and thiamin in fortified white rice are found on the outer layer of the grain, rinsing rice before cooking will wash these nutrients away. It's best to go straight from the bag into the cooking water, Negm says. The exception is when you're using imported rice, which may contain more impurities than the domestic kinds.

# Sea Vegetables
## PROTECTION FROM THE DEEP

When the Beatles were crooning "Octopus's Garden" back in 1969, they almost certainly weren't extolling the virtues of seaweed, or sea vegetables, as they're called by those who harvest and consume them today. But given what we've learned about these valuable plants, they probably should have been.

Eaten regularly, sea vegetables can be a valuable source of essential vitamins and minerals. In addition, they contain a variety of protective compounds that may help ward off some serious health threats, such as cancer.

## A TRADITIONAL CANCER-FIGHTER

For hundreds, maybe thousands of years, sea vegetables have been used in Asian cultures to prevent and treat cancer. As is often the case, research now indicates that there is more than a little scientific evidence supporting these ancient healing methods.

"We need more clinical studies, but so far there have been some interesting population and animal studies showing that sea vegetables can prevent tumors," says Alfred A. Bushway, Ph.D., professor of food science at the University of Maine in Orono, who believes that sea vegetables may be partially responsible for the lower cancer rates in countries like Japan, where the sea vegetable is as ubiquitous as our potato.

Japanese researchers studied the effects of extracts from eight different kinds of sea vegetables on cells that had been treated with potent cancer-causing agents. The results showed that sea vegetables may have tumor-squelching power.

Though scientists are unsure which compounds in sea vegetables are responsible, they suspect it may be beta-carotene, the same antioxidant compound found in such things as carrots and sweet potatoes. The sea vegetable called nori (also known as laver), which comes in dried sheets, is a good source of beta-carotene.

Researchers suspect that sea vegetables may have cancer-fighting compounds that simply aren't found in their land-loving counterparts. For example, a compound called sodium alginate, which is found in high concentrations in sea vegetables, could have cancer-fighting abilities, says Dr. Bushway. "But, again, this is a research area that needs to be more fully explored," he says.

## KELP FOR YOUR HEART AND BLOOD

If you want your blood to have the strength of the sea itself, a dose of vegetables from its waters can help.

One ounce of kelp, a thin, tender sea vegetable often used in soups and stir-fries, provides 51 micrograms, 13 percent of the Daily Value (DV) of folate, a nutrient that helps break down protein in the body and aids in the regeneration of red blood cells. An ounce of nori, the sea vegetable frequently used in sushi, provides 42 micrograms, 11 percent of the DV of this vital nutrient.

Kelp also contains magnesium, a mineral that has been found to keep high blood pressure in check, especially among people who are sensitive to sodium. One ounce of kelp has more than 34 milligrams, or almost 9 percent of the DV of this heart-healthy nutrient.

## A SEA OF IMMUNITY

You don't see too many whales swimming around with the sniffles. Maybe that's because of all the sea vegetables they're skimming off the ocean's swells.

Certain varieties of sea vegetables are packed with important vitamins that boost immunity and help fend off a host of diseases.

Topping this list is the nutritious nori. One ounce of raw nori contains 11 milligrams of infection-fighting vitamin C, more than 18 percent of the DV. Vitamin C is an antioxidant nutrient known for its ability to sweep up harmful, tissue-damaging oxygen molecules called free radicals.

An ounce of nori also delivers nearly 1,500 international units of vitamin A, 30 percent of the DV. Studies show that vitamin A not only builds immunity but also can safegaurd against night blindness and vision problems associated with aging, like macular degeneration. In addition, vitamin A can protect against several kinds of cancer.

## GOOD NEWS FOR VEGANS

If you're among the strictest of vegetarians, meaning that you don't eat meat, meat products, milk, or eggs, you may want to add some sea vegetables to your palette of land vegetables. It's a helpful way to ensure that you're getting adequate amounts of vitamin $B_{12}$, a nutrient most commonly found in meat.

Although there's some controversy about how much vitamin $B_{12}$ sea vegetables provide, experts agree that those who regularly dine on them have higher levels of vitamin $B_{12}$ in their blood than those who do not.

In one study of 21 strict vegetarians, researchers found that those who ate sea vegetables regularly had blood levels of vitamin $B_{12}$ twice as high as those who didn't eat the vegetables.

Without adequate amounts of vitamin $B_{12}$, you can experience fatigue, memory loss, and nerve damage resulting in tingling in the feet and hands. Although few people are at risk for vitamin $B_{12}$ deficiency, it can be a concern for strict vegetarians and for some elderly people who have trouble absorbing this vital nutrient.

# Getting the Most

**Rinse lightly.** Since many of the valuable trace minerals in dried sea vegetables are on the surface, experts recommend using a light touch when rinsing them prior to cooking. "Some people soak and rinse the life out of their sea vegetables," says Dr. Bushway. "We just recommend light rinsing. Otherwise you'll lose a lot of the surface minerals, like potassium."

**Invest in stock.** The best way to retain the maximum amount of nutrients is to make soup out of your sea vegetables, says Dr. Bushway. "When sea vegetables are used in soups, some of the minerals are released in the broth," he says. "The remainder provide valuable fiber and unique phytochemicals, such as the alginate found in kelp."

**Eat for variety.** It doesn't take a lot of sea vegetables to get the benefits. "Nutritional studies indicate that as little as $1/4$ ounce of dried sea vegetables can make a significant nutritional contribution to your diet," says Dr. Bushway.

The best way to include more sea vegetables in your diet is to experiment. "Add small, bite-size pieces to salads, soups, stews, grain dishes, stir-fries, and sandwiches," says Carl Karush of Maine Coast Sea Vegetables in Franklin.

# Shellfish

## HEALTH FROM THE SEA

For most folks, shellfish like lobster, shrimp, scallops, and oysters are luxuries—foods to be reserved for special occasions. For one thing, shellfish are expensive, often costing twice as much (or more) as other fish. Shellfish also have a reputation for containing boatloads of cholesterol and a sea of sodium, both of which health-conscious diners usually try to avoid.

While it's true that shellfish are high in cholesterol and sodium, these aren't the health threats that scientists once thought they were, says Robert M. Grodner, Ph.D., professor emeritus in the department of food science at Louisiana State University in Baton Rouge. In addition, shellfish contain generous amounts of vitamins, minerals, and other healthful compounds that more than offset their slight nutritional downside.

### GOOD FOR THE HEART

Ironically, the very thing that makes shellfish so healthful is the same stuff most of us are trying to avoid: the fat. Yet the kind of fat found in shellfish, known as omega-3 fatty acids, is very good for the heart. Researchers at the University of Washington in Seattle found that people who ate enough seafood to get almost 6 grams of omega-3's a month had half the risk of cardiac arrest, an often fatal irregularity in heart rhythm, of those who ate none.

In fact, people who eat a lot of seafood fare even better than vegetarians when it comes to heart health. In one study, seafood-eaters with high concentrations of omega-3's in their blood had significantly lower blood pressure and lower levels of cholesterol and triglycerides—blood fats that in large amounts can increase the risk of heart disease—than vegetarians who didn't eat shellfish. Although many of the studies on omega-3's have focused on fish like salmon and mackerel, all fish, including shellfish, contain some omega-3's, says Dan Sharp, M.D., Ph.D., director of the Honolulu Heart Program.

The omega-3's in shellfish have a number of benefits. They strengthen the heart muscle, enabling it to beat steadily and soundly. They help lower blood pressure, keep cholesterol in check, and also reduce the tendency of platelets—tiny discs in the blood—from sticking together and causing clots.

Atlantic and Pacific oysters are particularly rich sources of omega-3's. Eating six medium oysters five to seven times a month will provide all the omega-3's your heart needs.

## MULTIVITAMINS IN A SHELL

Aside from their role in protecting the heart, shellfish are incredibly rich sources of a variety of essential (and hard-to-find) vitamins and minerals. Shellfish contain large amounts of vitamin $B_{12}$, for example, which the body uses to keep nerves healthy and make red blood cells. When levels of vitamin $B_{12}$ slip, the body (and mind) can literally short-circuit, causing memory loss, confusion, slow reflexes, and fatigue. In fact, what's sometimes thought to be senility in older people is sometimes nothing more than a lack of vitamin $B_{12}$.

Three ounces of crab contains 10 micrograms of vitamin $B_{12}$, 167 percent of the Daily Value (DV). Clams are even better, with 3 ounces—about nine small steamed clams—providing 1,400 percent of the DV.

With the exception of shrimp, shellfish also contain a lot of zinc, which is essential for keeping the immune system strong. Oysters are the best source, with six oysters containing about 27 milligrams, almost 181 percent of the DV.

It's sometimes hard to get enough iron from foods, which is why about 20 percent of Americans are low in this important mineral. But if you can muster up enough muscle to lift a mussel to your mouth, you'll get much of the iron you need to help prevent iron-deficiency anemia. Three ounces of mussels provides about 6 milligrams of iron, 60 percent of the Recommended Dietary Allowance (RDA) for men and 40 percent of the RDA for women. Clams are an even better source, with nine small clams containing about 24 milligrams of iron, 240 percent of the RDA for men and 160 percent of the RDA for women.

Finally, many shellfish are good sources of magnesium, potassium, and vitamin C. The vitamin C is a great bonus because it helps the body absorb more of the iron found in these foods.

## A New Reputation

Although people are often nervous about eating shellfish because these foods contain large amounts of sodium and cholesterol, neither of these items is likely to cause problems for most folks.

For one thing, even though 3 ounces of shellfish contains between 50 and 170 milligrams of cholesterol (depending on the type of shellfish), the cholesterol found in food is unlikely to have a serious effect on cholesterol in the body. "Unlike other cholesterol sources, such as red meat, shellfish contain almost no saturated fat," explains Dr. Grodner. Eating a diet high in saturated fat is much more likely to send your cholesterol soaring than eating the cholesterol itself, he says.

Then there's the sodium. As you would expect of creatures from the sea, shellfish contain quite a bit—about 150 to 900 milligrams in a 3-ounce serving, depending on the type. But unless your doctor has suggested that you reduce the amount of salt in your diet, shellfish shouldn't be a problem. One serving of shellfish is well within the DV of 2,400 milligrams of sodium.

# Getting the Most

**Eat them with vitamin C.** Since your body is better able to absorb the iron in foods when you eat them with vitamin C, it's a good idea to include vitamin C–rich foods such as broccoli or peppers on the shellfish menu.

**Mix and match.** Because shellfish are usually considered a luxury item, most people eat only a handful or two at a time. An easy way to include more of them in your diet is to toss them together in one big, briny stew, says Dr. Grodner. "It can be a mighty healthful meal," he says.

# Soy Foods
## HELP FOR YOUR HORMONES

In a perfect world, milkshakes would lower cholesterol, burgers would help prevent cancer, and cheesecake would ease hot flashes, mood swings, and other uncomfortable conditions associated with menopause.

Sound far-fetched? Maybe not—if they were made with soy. According to researchers, all of these health benefits and more have been linked to this small bean that many Americans have never seen, let alone eaten—the common soybean.

Studies show that several compounds found in soybeans and in related foods like tofu, tempeh, and soy milk may help lower cholesterol, reduce the risk of heart disease and cancer, and ease some of the discomfort of menopause. Indeed, if early research proves fruitful, women in the future may use soy foods as a replacement for, or at least as a supplement to, estrogen replacement therapy.

Researchers speculate that the key to soy's healing power is a class of compounds called phytoestrogens. Phytoestrogens such as genistein and daidzein are weaker versions of the estrogen women produce naturally. They appear to help in a number of different ways, from blocking the negative effects of natural estrogens to supplementing them when they're running low.

Evidence of soy's health benefits is still preliminary, experts warn. Nonetheless, the possibilities are intriguing. "The data emerging on soy are really exciting," says James W. Anderson, M.D., professor of medicine and clinical nutrition at the Veterans Administration Medical Center at the University of Kentucky College of Medicine in Lexington and one of the nation's leading fiber researchers.

With Americans becoming more and more aware of this lowly legume's healing powers, some grocery stores have begun stocking a wide variety of soy foods, from soy-protein shakes and tempeh burgers to tofu cheesecake.

## GOOD FOR YOUR HEART

You know that high cholesterol is a major risk factor for heart disease. Putting more soy foods in your diet may play a role in sending cholesterol levels south.

As proof of the benefits of soy, researchers point to Asian countries, where people eat tofu, tempeh, or other soy foods virtually every day. Consider the Japanese: They live longer than people anywhere else in the world. Japanese men have the world's lowest rate of death from heart disease, with Japanese women coming in a close second. A possible reason is that the Japanese eat about 24 pounds of soy foods per person per year, which averages about 1 ounce a day. Americans, by contrast, eat an average of 4 pounds per person per year.

Researchers speculate that soy foods increase the activity of low-density lipoprotein (LDL) cholesterol receptors, "traps" on the surfaces of cells that seize harmful LDL molecules from the bloodstream and ship them to the liver, from which they're eventually excreted. Reducing the amount of LDL in the blood may help keep it from oxidizing and clogging the arteries leading from the heart.

In one large study, Dr. Anderson and his colleagues analyzed the results of 38 separate studies examining the relationship between soy and cholesterol levels. Their conclusion: Consuming 1 to 1½ ounces of soy protein (rather than animal protein) a day lowered total cholesterol by 9 percent and harmful LDL cholesterol by 13 percent. As a bonus, the levels of "good" high-density lipoprotein (HDL) cholesterol weren't reduced by the soy. Other studies support Dr. Anderson's analysis. Researchers at the University of Illinois at Urbana-Champaign gave 21 men with high cholesterol two types of muffins. Some muffins contained soy protein and fiber. Others had fiber alone. Men who consumed the soy-protein muffins had significantly lower total cholesterol than men eating the fiber-only muffins.

## TURNING DOWN THE HEAT

More than half of American women in menopause complain of hot flashes and night sweats. In Japan, by contrast, there isn't even a phrase for "hot flash." Might Japanese women have fewer menopausal problems because they eat more soy?

"There are some preliminary data that suggest that soy reduces menopause symptoms such as hot flashes," says Mark Messina, Ph.D., former head of the National Cancer Institute's Designer Foods Program.

In one study, researchers at the Brighton Medical Clinic in Victoria, Australia, gave 58 postmenopausal women about 1$^1$/$_2$ ounces of soy flour or wheat flour every day. After three months, the women eating soy flour saw their hot flashes plummet by 40 percent. Women given wheat flour, by contrast, had only a 25 percent reduction.

"If these data are confirmed, then within a couple of years we may be at a point where doctors are saying, 'Take 2 cups of soy milk per day' instead of recommending hormone replacement therapy to relieve menopause symptoms," says Dr. Messina.

## POWERFUL BREAST PROTECTION

Researchers believe that the phytoestrogens in soy, which mimic a woman's natural estrogen, may help reduce the effects of the hormone in the body. Since estrogen is thought to fuel the growth of breast tumors, lower activity in the body could mean a lower risk of developing breast cancer.

The estrogens in soy can help protect women in several ways, depending on the stage of life. In premenopausal women, for example, a diet high in soy foods may lengthen the menstrual cycle. This is important, since every woman experiences a surge in estrogen at the beginning of her cycle. Multiplied over a lifetime, these surges expose the body to large amounts of estrogen, which eventually could cause cellular changes that lead to cancer. Lengthening the menstrual cycle, experts say, reduces the frequency of these surges, and with it a woman's lifetime exposure to the hormone.

In one study, researchers at the National University of Singapore found that premenopausal women who consumed high amounts of soy foods, along with generous amounts of beta-carotene and polyunsaturated fats, had half the risk of developing breast cancer as women who consumed a lot of animal protein.

Curiously, in women who are postmenopausal, soy foods appear to provide an estrogen "lift" that helps make up for the body's low levels of the hormone. What's more, this lift appears to provide the protective benefits of estrogen (such as helping to prevent osteoporosis) without raising the cancer risk.

## PROTECTION FOR MEN

While most research exploring the protective effects of soy foods has looked at women, experts agree that men can benefit as well.

It appears that a soy-rich diet may help reduce the harmful effects of the male hormone testosterone, which is thought to fuel the growth of cancerous cells in the prostate gland.

A study of 8,000 Japanese men living in Hawaii found that those who ate the most tofu had the lowest rates of prostate cancer. Even though Japanese men develop prostate cancer just as often as Western men do, they nonetheless have the lowest death rates from prostate cancer in the world. Experts suspect that soy foods, by inhibiting the effects of testosterone, help shut off the "fuel" that causes cancers to grow.

For both men and women, "what these studies suggest is that just one serving is enough to reduce cancer risk," says Dr. Messina. "If that's for real, then soy could have a tremendous public health impact."

### NUTRITIONAL EXTRAS

There's more to tofu, tempeh, and other soy foods than phytoestrogens. Soy foods are just plain good for you. "There are lots of reasons to add soy to your diet just from a basic nutritional perspective," says Dr. Messina.

For example, a half-cup of tofu provides about 20 grams of protein, 40 percent of the Daily Value (DV). The same half-cup supplies about 258 milligrams of calcium, more than 25 percent of the DV, and 13 milligrams of iron, 87 percent of the Recommended Dietary Allowance (RDA) for women and 130 percent of the RDA for men.

While soy foods are moderately high in fat, most of the fat is polyunsaturated. Soy foods contain little of the artery-clogging saturated fat that is found in meats and many dairy foods, says Dr. Messina. So you can feel good about eating soy foods without worrying about the fat.

## Getting the Most

**Add it last.** When cooking with tofu, tempeh, or other soy products, always add them late in the cooking process. Researchers speculate that cooking at high heats for extended periods of time may reduce or eliminate many of the nutritional benefits. "Overcooking may leach out the phytoestrogen content," says Dr. Anderson.

**Shop for power.** While it's best to eat soy foods in their unadulterated form, there are times that you may have a taste for a ready-made vegetable burger or breakfast sausage. When buying processed soy foods, make sure that they contain "soy protein," "hydrolyzed vegetable protein," or "textured vegetable protein," which are all acceptable sources of phytoestrogens. By contrast, don't expect too much from products containing soy protein concentrates, says Dr. Anderson. "Unfortunately, most of the beneficial substances are extracted from these products," he says.

**Look for full-fat.** While it's usually a good idea to reduce the amount of fat in your diet, full-fat soy milk contains 50 percent more phytoestrogens than the low-fat kind, says Dr. Anderson. "Getting those extra phytoestrogens is a good trade-off for the extra fat," he says.

# Squash

## THE GOURDS OF LIFE

Judging from remains found in Mexican caves, folks have been eating squash for 7,000 years. Squash was one of the nourishing "three sisters" in early Native American diets. (The other two were corn and beans.) And they were considered so important that they were buried with the dead to feed them on their final journey.

It has taken science a few thousand years to prove what early Americans knew from experience: Squash is almost overloaded with nourishing compounds, so much so that scientists have just begun to map its healing potential. "I don't think anybody really knows all the good substances there are in squash," says Dexter L. Morris, M.D., Ph.D., vice chairman and associate professor in the department of emergency medicine at the University of North Carolina School of Medicine at Chapel Hill.

When researchers talk about the healing powers of squash, what they're usually referring to is winter squash such as hubbard, acorn, and butternut, which are distinguished by their deep yellow and orange flesh colors. Pale summer squash, by contrast, while low in calories and a decent source of fiber, is generally regarded as a nutritional lightweight, at least unless future research proves otherwise.

"Not long ago I was saying that apples and onions didn't have much in them," admits Mark Kestin, Ph.D., chairman of the nutrition program at Bastyr University and affiliate associate professor of epidemiology at the University of Washington School of Medicine, both in Seattle. Then researchers discovered heart-saving flavonoids, and the produce suddenly looked rich. "Summer squash may have some incredible substance we haven't discovered yet," he says.

## COLOR THEM HEALTHY

The winter squash come in an enormous variety of shapes and textures, ranging from baby acorn squash the size of a walnut to huge hubbards as big as a bowling pin. Yet there's one thing that they all have in common: strong, intense colors that indicate the presence of healing compounds within.

Two of the most popular winter squashes, the bumpy-skinned hubbard squash and the deeply tanned butternut squash, are both rich in vitamin C and beta-carotene, two antioxidant vitamins that have been shown in studies to help prevent cancer, heart disease, and certain age-related conditions such as problems with the eyes. Eating a half-cup of baked butternut squash will provide more than a quarter of the Daily Value (DV) for vitamin C. The same amount of squash delivers 40 to 66 percent of the amount of beta-carotene recommended by experts.

For people with asthma, squash and other foods rich in vitamin C can be powerful breath savers. It's easy to understand why. Modern life is filled with car exhaust, cigarette smoke, and other pollutants—scientists call them oxidants—that can weaken our lungs. Foods like squash, however, are rich in antioxidants, like vitamin C. Studies have shown that the more vitamin C you get, the lower your risk of getting asthma or other respiratory diseases.

"People who have more C in their diets over time have fewer lung ailments. The vitamin gets transported to the lining of the lung and serves as an antioxidant there," explains Gary E. Hatch, Ph.D., research toxicologist in the pulmonary toxicology branch of the Environmental Protection Agency.

Dr. Hatch recommends that everyone get at least 200 milligrams daily of dietary vitamin C, which is about the amount in $6^1/2$ cups of baked butternut squash.

On the beta-carotene front, "there are tons of studies showing that eating vegetables rich in beta-carotene" is good for you, says Dr. Morris. Doctors in Italy and Switzerland studied the diets of more than 1,000 of their countrywomen. Preliminary research suggests that women who got the most beta-carotene—5.5 milligrams a day, which is about the amount in 1 cup of baked winter squash—had half the risk of endometrial cancer of those who ate the least.

# Getting the Most

**Shop for color.** There's a huge variability in the amount of beta-carotene found in squash. It can range anywhere from about 0.5 milligram to about 5 milligrams, even in the same kind of squash. As a rule, experts say, the darker the squash, the more beta-carotene.

The shell of an acorn squash, for example, should be an intensely dark green. Butternut squash should be a butterscotch tan, and hubbards should be almost glow-in-the-dark orange.

"The richer the color, the richer the nutrient content," says Susan Thom, R.D., a resource spokesperson for the American Dietetic Association and a nutrition consultant in Brecksville, Ohio.

**Buy it ahead of time.** The hard skin that makes winter squash so tough to cut also protects the flesh inside. This means that you can store it for a month or more in a cool, well-ventilated place before the nutrients start to diminish. In fact, storing squash actually causes the amount of beta-carotene to increase, according to Densie Webb, R.D., Ph.D., co-author of *Foods for Better Health*.

**Try the summer kind.** While zucchini and other kinds of summer squash don't have the rich nutrient stores of winter squash, they do contain a lot of fiber, but only if you eat the peel, says Pamela Savage-Marr, R.D., a spokesperson for the American Dietetic Association and a health education specialist at Oakwood Health Care System in Dearborn, Michigan. A half-cup of unpeeled, uncooked summer squash contains more than 1 gram of fiber.

# Sweet Peppers

## PICK A PECK FOR HEALTH

Peter Piper wasn't the only person who picked peppers. So did Christopher Columbus, who brought sweet peppers, along with news that the world wasn't flat, from the Americas back to Spain, where they quickly became an integral part of the cuisine.

Due to the growing interest in ethnic cuisines, sweet peppers, which range in color from dark green to fire engine red, depending on how long they're left on the vine, aren't found only in salad bars anymore. They're also being used in soups, sauces, purees, and pasta dishes. Peppers do more than add a sweet high note to recipes. They're also filled with nutrients that have been shown to battle cataracts and heart disease. And unlike their fiery-tempered siblings, the chili peppers, sweet peppers are mild enough to eat in large amounts, so you can easily reap their health benefits.

### STUFFED WITH ANTIOXIDANTS

Even though sweet peppers such as bell peppers, pimientos, and frying peppers don't get as much attention as broccoli, cauliflower, and other powerhouse foods, they're among the most nutrient-dense vegetables you can buy, especially when it comes to vitamin C and beta-carotene. (As a rule, the redder the pepper, the more beta-carotene it contains.)

Bite for bite, few vegetables contain as much beta-carotene (which is converted to vitamin A in the body) as the sweet red pepper. This is important because beta-carotene plays a key role in keeping the immune system healthy. It's also a potent antioxidant, meaning that it fights tissue-damaging oxygen molecules known as free radicals, which scientists believe contribute to major health foes like cataracts and heart disease.

Sweet red peppers are such a good source of beta-carotene that a group of German researchers has classified them as a "must-eat" food for people trying to get more of this important antioxidant. One pepper provides 4 milligrams of beta-carotene, 40 to 66 percent of the recommended daily amount of 6 to 10 milligrams.

Both sweet red and green peppers also contain generous amounts of vitamin C, another powerful antioxidant. A half-cup of chopped green pepper (about half a pepper) contains 45 milligrams of vitamin C, 74 percent of the Daily Value (DV). Sweet red peppers are even better, with the same-size serving providing 142 milligrams of vitamin C, 236 percent of the DV. That's more than twice the amount that you'd get from a medium-size orange.

The combination of vitamin C and beta-carotene can provide potent protection against cataracts. In a study of more than 900 people, Italian researchers found that those who ate sweet peppers and other foods rich in beta-carotene regularly were significantly less likely to have cataracts than those who did not.

The only problem with sweet peppers is that their nutrient content varies with the environment they're grown in, says Paul Bosland, Ph.D., professor in the department of horticulture at New Mexico State University in Las Cruces and founder of the Chile Pepper Institute at the university. You're best off buying peppers that are grown in optimum conditions, where the temperature is about 68°F all the time, because they have the most beta-carotene," he says. That means the most nutritious peppers are generally available during their peak growing season from July to September. Meanwhile, scientists are trying to develop a strain of peppers that's consistently high in these vital nutrients.

## Getting the Most

**Cook them lightly.** Since vitamin C is fragile, it's readily destroyed during cooking. Eating peppers raw will provide the most of this nutrient. Beta-carotene, on the other hand, needs a little heat to release it from the pepper's fiber cells. To get the most of both nutrients, it's a good idea to steam, sauté, or microwave peppers until they're done but still have a little crunch.

**Add some fat.** In order for beta-carotene to be absorbed into the bloodstream, it needs to be accompanied by a little fat. Drizzling peppers with a touch of oil, before or after cooking, will help you get the most of this important compound. If you're eating raw peppers, dunking them in a bit of dip will also help the beta-carotene be absorbed.

**Mix 'em up.** Even though peppers are one of the healthiest vegetables going, few people eat enough of them to get the full benefit. The easiest way to get more peppers in your diet is to use them as an ingredient in other foods, says Dr. Bosland. You can use peppers to add a sweet punch to foods such as pasta, tuna salad, and green salad, for example.

**Raise a glassful.** Another way to get more peppers in your diet is to make them into juice. The juice from two green peppers contains 132 milligrams of vitamin C, three times the amount you'd get from the usual half-cup serving. Although pepper juice isn't very appetizing on its own, it adds a sweet zip to other juices, such as carrot juice. Try mixing four or five carrots with two green bell peppers in a juicer for a supercharged antioxidant cocktail.

# Tea

## A CUP OF GOOD HEALTH

What would you think if a man in a string tie and a long, black coat came up to you and said, "Psss-ss-st. Wanna buy a drink that stops cancer of the skin, lung, stomach, colon, liver, breast, esophagus, and pancreas? And cancer of the small intestine? And heart disease and strokes? And cavities—did I say cavities?"

"Snake oil salesman": That's what you'd think.

Well, Mister Snake Oil would be more right than wrong. Laboratory studies have shown that tea has indeed stopped tumors from forming. The risk of stroke and heart disease tumbles when you drink tea. And tea does have clout against cavities.

Tea contains hundreds of compounds called polyphenols. These compounds act like antioxidants—that is, they help neutralize harmful oxygen molecules in the body known as free radicals, which have been linked to cancer, heart disease, and a number of less serious problems, such as wrinkles.

"In general, polyphenols are very, very good antioxidants. But the best polyphenols are in tea, which has a lot of them," says Joe A. Vinson, Ph.D., professor of chemistry at the University of Scranton in Pennsylvania. "They make up nearly 30 percent of tea's dry weight."

This may help explain why tea is the most popular beverage in the world.

### ARTERIAL PROTECTION

Blocked arteries, and the heart attacks, high blood pressure, and strokes they can lead to, don't happen all at once. They're typically preceded by years of steadily increasing damage, in which the body's dangerous low-density lipoprotein (LDL) cholesterol oxidizes and gradually clings to artery walls, making them stiff and narrow.

That's where tea can help. In studies, Dr. Vinson found that the

polyphenols found in tea were extremely effective in preventing cholesterol from oxidizing and fouling blood vessels. In fact, one of the
polyphenols in tea, epigallocatechin gallate, was able to neutralize five
times as much LDL cholesterol as vitamin C, the strongest of the antioxidant vitamins.

One reason that tea's polyphenols are so effective is that they can
work in two places at once, blocking the harmful effects of oxidized
LDL cholesterol both in the bloodstream and at the artery walls,
"where LDL really produces atherosclerosis," says Dr. Vinson.

In a Dutch study of 800 men, researchers found that those who ate
the most flavonoids, a large chemical family that includes tea's
polyphenols, had a 58 percent lower risk of dying from heart disease
than those who ate the least. When the results were further analyzed,
it was revealed that the healthiest men were those getting more than
half their flavonoids from black tea, with onions and apples con-
tributing most of the rest.

You don't need to drink rivers of tea to get the benefits. In the
Dutch study the healthiest men drank about 4 cups of tea a day.

Just as tea helps protect arteries leading from the heart, it has a similar effect on those in or leading to the brain, says Dr. Vinson.

In another large study, Dutch researchers looked at the diets of 550
men ages 50 to 69. As in the heart study, men with the highest
flavonoid levels—those who drank almost 5 cups of black tea a day or
more—were 69 percent less likely to have a stroke than the men who
drank less than 3 cups a day.

## HELP AGAINST CANCER

Every time you fry a hamburger or broil a pork chop, compounds
called heterocyclic amines form on the surface of the food. In the body
these chemicals turn into more dangerous forms, which can cause
cancer, says John H. Weisburger, Ph.D., senior member of the American Health Foundation in Valhalla, New York.

"Data suggest that because of eating fried or broiled meat, the
Western population has a significantly elevated risk of intestinal
cancer," he says.

Enter the tea polyphenols. Inside the body these compounds help
prevent the formation of potential carcinogens, Dr. Weisburger says.
In other words, they help stop cancer before it starts.

In experiments at Case Western University School of Medicine in
Cleveland, Hasan Mukhtar, Ph.D., professor of dermatology and en-

vironmental health sciences, has seen tea stop cancer at each stage of its life cycle, arresting both its growth and spread. And where cancerous tumors have already formed, he has seen tea shrink them.

Studying the effects of green tea on sunburned skin in laboratory animals, Dr. Mukhtar found that the animals given tea developed one-tenth as many tumors as those given water. (Even when the tea-treated animals developed tumors, they were often benign, not cancerous.) What's more, tea was equally effective whether given as a drink or applied to the skin. Some cosmetics companies have started adding green tea to skin products for its potential protective benefits.

Dr. Mukhtar believes the polyphenols in tea can act even earlier, possibly keeping DNA, the very substance of our cells, strong and healthy and less likely to cause the cell to change into a cancer cell.

### Good for the Teeth

Having a toothache generally isn't a big deal, unless it's your toothache. Tea can help prevent the pain, since it contains numerous compounds, polyphenols as well as tannin, that act as antibiotics. In other words, tea is great for mopping up bacteria that promote tooth decay.

Tea also contains fluoride, which provides further dental protection. When researchers at Forsyth Dental Center in Boston tested a variety of foods for their antibacterial qualities, they found that tea was far and away the most protective.

Japanese researchers at Kyushu University in Fukuoka, Japan, have identified four components in tea—tannin, catechin, caffeine, and tocopherol (a vitamin E–like substance)—that help increase the acid resistance of tooth enamel. This quartet of compounds was made even more effective with the addition of extra fluoride. The extra oomph made tooth enamel 98 percent impervious to the action of acids on the teeth.

## Getting the Most

**Steep three and see.** When you brew tea, it takes 3 minutes for it to release the health-promoting compounds. That's also the amount of time researchers use in their studies on tea. Although longer steeping causes more compounds to be released, "those compounds are bitter. And a bigger dose doesn't necessarily put twice as much of them in the body," says Dr. Vinson.

**Bag it.** Tea aficionados always use loose tea. No easy tea bags for them. But the pulverized contents of tea bags actually release more polyphenols than the larger loose leaves. That's because the tiny particles in the bag yield more surface area for polyphenols to dissolve into hot water.

**Pick your flavors.** Although green tea has been more thoroughly researched than the black variety (mainly because the first studies were done in China and Japan, where green tea is the preferred brew), both kinds show equally salutary effects, says Dr. Vinson.

If you prefer decaffeinated tea, by all means drink up. The removal of caffeine has little effect on tea's polyphenol content, so little is lost in the translation, Dr. Vinson says.

The same goes for bottled teas, iced tea, and teas made from mixes, Dr. Vinson adds. In fact, some soft drink and juice companies have been so impressed with tea's benefits that they've begun fortifying their beverages with green tea. Check out your health food store for new products.

**Hold the milk—at least for now.** One preliminary study in Italy found that adding milk to tea, as the British do at tea time, blocked tea's antioxidant benefits.

"There is some evidence that milk protein binds to some of the tea compounds and blocks their absorption. But those compounds could get unbound in the stomach. So we're not so sure milk is bad," says Dr. Vinson.

**Keep it fresh.** If you make your own iced tea, drink it within a few days, suggests Dr. Vinson. "And make sure you cover it to keep it fresh when you refrigerate it," he advises. "My experience tells me not to keep iced tea for more than a week because the concentration of compounds falls off. You get to the point where about 10 percent has been lost or changed."

**Have tea with meat.** Since tea's polyphenol compounds help block the formation of cancer-causing chemicals, it's a good idea to enjoy a tea party after eating fried or broiled meat. A meat-eater's rule of thumb: Whenever you eat fried meat, have a couple of cups of tea at the same time.

# Tomatoes

## PREVENTION FROM THE GARDEN

If it weren't for Colonel Robert Gibbon Johnson, Americans might never have tasted tomatoes.

For centuries tomatoes, which are members of the deadly nightshade family, were thought to be toxic, capable of causing appendicitis, cancer, and "brain fever." But Colonel Johnson, an admittedly eccentric gentleman, thought otherwise. After a trip overseas in the early 1800s, he returned to Salem, New Jersey, with tomatoes and a plan to liberate this lush, red fruit from its fearsome reputation.

Never one to miss a dramatic opportunity, Johnson announced to the townsfolk that on September 26, 1820, he would eat not one but an entire basket of tomatoes. Public excitement was high, and some 2,000 spectators arrived to watch Johnson commit what they were certain would be suicide.

He lived, of course, and tomatoes went on to become our favorite fruit. Indeed, Americans eat more tomatoes, both fresh and processed, than nearly any other fruit or vegetable. It's a good thing, too, because tomatoes contain compounds that can help prevent a number of serious conditions, from heart disease and cancer to cataracts.

## CELLULAR PROTECTION

Tomatoes contain a red pigment called lycopene. This compound appears to act as an antioxidant—that is, it helps neutralize cell-damaging oxygen molecules called free radicals before they cause damage.

Until recently, lycopene's reputation for healing was overshadowed by its well-studied cousin, beta-carotene. But newer studies indicate that lycopene could have twice the cancer-fighting punch of beta-carotene.

In one large study of nearly 48,000 men, Harvard researchers found that men who ate at least 10 servings a week of tomatoes, whether raw, cooked, or in sauce, were able to cut their risk of developing prostate cancer by 45 percent. Ten servings sounds like a lot, but when they're spread out over an entire week, it's probably not much more than you're getting now. A single serving, after all, is only a half-cup of tomato sauce or the sauce on a slice of pizza.

"Lycopene is a very strong antioxidant," says Meir Stampfer, M.D., co-author of the study and professor of epidemiology and nutrition at the Harvard School of Public Health. "For some reason lycopene concentrates in the prostate. Men with high levels of lycopene in their blood are at lower risk for prostate cancer."

The benefits of tomatoes aren't limited to the prostate gland. In laboratory studies Israeli researchers found that lycopene is also a powerful inhibitor of breast, lung, and endometrial cancer cells.

Almost no one reaps more benefits from tomatoes than Italians, who eat them in one form or another virtually every day. Researchers in Italy found that people who ate seven or more servings of raw tomatoes a week had a 60 percent lower chance of developing stomach, colon, or rectal cancers than folks who ate two servings or less. Once again, lycopene is thought to account for at least some of the protective effects.

Research also suggests that getting more lycopene in the diet may help older people stay active longer. In a study of 88 nuns ages 77 to 98, researchers found that those who got the most lycopene were the ones least likely to need help with daily activities such as getting dressed and walking.

## New Discoveries

In the not-too-distant future, doctors may be recommending tomatoes as a way of preventing lung cancer. Tomatoes contain two powerful compounds, coumaric acid and chlorogenic acid, that may help block the effects of nitrosamines, which are cancer-causing compounds that form naturally in the body and "are the most potent carcinogen in tobacco smoke," says Joseph Hotchkiss, Ph.D., professor of food chemistry and toxicology at Cornell University in Ithaca, New York.

Until recently, scientists believed that it was the vitamin C in fruits and vegetables that helped neutralize these dangerous compounds. But a study conducted by Dr. Hotchkiss and his colleagues revealed that tomatoes blocked the formation of nitrosamines even after the vitamin C was removed.

The protective coumaric and chlorogenic acids found in tomatoes are also found in other fruits and vegetables, like carrots, green peppers, pineapples, and strawberries. Dr. Hotchkiss speculates that these compounds may be one of the reasons that people who eat more fruits and vegetables have a lower risk of developing cancer.

## ADDITIONAL PROTECTION

It's not only lemons and limes that are high in vitamin C. Tomatoes also contain loads of this powerful vitamin, which has been shown to help relieve conditions ranging from cataracts and cancer to heart disease. One medium-size tomato provides almost 24 milligrams, or 40 percent of the Daily Value (DV) for vitamin C.

Tomatoes are also a good source of vitamin A, a vitamin that has been shown to boost immunity and help prevent cancer. One medium tomato provides 766 international units of vitamin A, 15 percent of the DV. In addition, a tomato provides 273 milligrams of potassium, 8 percent of the DV. They also have about 1 gram of iron, 7 percent of the Recommended Dietary Allowance (RDA) for women and 10 percent of the RDA for men. While the amount of iron is small, your body absorbs it very efficiently when it's taken with vitamin C, which tomatoes have in abundance.

# Getting the Most

**Shop for color.** When buying fresh tomatoes, look for a brilliant shade of red. Red, ripe tomatoes can have four times more beta-carotene than green, immature ones.

**Shop for convenience.** You don't have to buy fresh tomatoes—or those pale impostors that hit the supermarket come February—to get healing benefits. Lycopene can withstand the high heats used in processing, so canned tomatoes and tomato sauce both contain their full complement of this helpful compound.

**Cook them a bit.** The lycopene in tomatoes is located in the cell walls. Cooking tomatoes in a little bit of oil causes the cell walls to burst, releasing more of the healing lycopene.

**Have a little fat.** "If you eat a tomato with a little bit of fat, like olive oil, you'll absorb the lycopene better," says Dr. Stampfer.

# Water

## FLUID FOR LIFE

Run your car without water in the radiator and it will come to a steaming halt. Yet people who wouldn't dream of letting their cars run dry often walk around without enough water in their own radiators. And because every cell in the body requires fluids to dissolve and transport vitamins, minerals, sugar, and other chemicals, not drinking enough water can leave you feeling like a run-down Ford.

The average person loses about 2 percent of her body weight (about 1½ quarts of water) in urine, perspiration, and other body fluids every day. To replace these fluids, doctors advise drinking at least eight glasses of water, milk, or juice a day—more if you're a large person, over age 55, sick with a cold, or simply active.

To make sure you drink enough, the brain has special sensors in a part of the brain called the thalamus, which monitor blood levels of sodium. When concentrations of sodium rise, it means that water levels are running low. The brain then sends a signal, in the form of thirst, that says it's time to head to the water cooler.

This system usually works well. As we age, however, the thirst sensor gets less sensitive, so we don't always drink enough, says Lucia Kaiser, R.D., Ph.D., assistant professor of nutrition and cooperative extension specialist at the University of California, Davis. Plus, sometimes we get so busy we simply don't take time to drink. And that can cause serious problems, ranging from kidney stones and constipation to fatigue. Let's take a look at a few of the ways in which water can keep you healthy.

### STOPPING STONES

Men say it's the worst pain they've ever known. Women say they'd rather have the pain of childbirth. Both men and women agree that once you've had a kidney stone, you never want to get another one.

Getting enough water, doctors say, will help ensure you never do. Normally, many of the wastes in the body are dissolved in fluids and carried out in the urine. But when you don't drink enough water, the wastes may become concentrated, forming crystals that can bond together and form kidney stones.

"I tell people to think of the insides of their bodies as they would their kitchens," says Bernell Baldwin, Ph.D., applied physiologist at Wildwood Lifestyle Center and Hospital in Georgia and science editor of *Journal of Health and Healing*. "You can't expect your body to be able to clean up its dishes without giving it enough water."

Here's an easy test to tell if you're getting enough water. Look at your urine. Except in the morning, when you haven't had fluids all night, it should be pale yellow or even clear. If it's dark, that means wastes are too concentrated and you should be drinking more water.

## FLUID MOVEMENTS

Another way in which water helps remove wastes from the body is by keeping the stools soft, which helps prevent constipation, says Dr. Baldwin. When you don't drink enough, stools become hard and dry, and it takes longer for them to move through your system.

Constipation isn't merely uncomfortable, Dr. Baldwin adds. Studies have shown that constipation may lead to other problems, such as hemorrhoids, diverticular disease, or even colon cancer.

"You should drink two glasses of water about a half-hour before eating breakfast," Dr. Baldwin advises. "This not only hydrates your body but also primes your system, flushing out wastes and getting it ready for food."

## WASH AWAY FATIGUE

We think of fatigue as being caused by not getting enough sleep or working too hard. But in many cases, the problem is even more basic: not getting enough water.

Here's what happens. When you don't drink enough, cells throughout your body start getting a little dry. To quench their thirst, they draw water from the most convenient place—the bloodstream. This leaves the blood thick, sludgy, and harder to pump. The extra work involved in pumping the blood can cause energy levels to decline, Dr. Baldwin says.

You don't have to run completely dry to feel the effects. In a small study of cyclists, researchers found that their performance levels dropped when they lost as little as 2 percent of their body weight in fluids—the equivalent of about six glasses of water.

## WASH AWAY WEIGHT

One of the nicest benefits of drinking more water is that it can help you lose weight. For one thing, many of us think it's time to eat when, in fact, we're merely thirsty. Drinking water is a great way to quell hunger pangs. In addition, when you drink with meals, you're more likely to take in fewer calories, says Dr. Kaiser.

Water can help in yet another way. When you drink cold water (40°F or cooler) you actually burn calories, because the body has to raise the temperature of the water to 98.6°F. In the process, it burns slightly less than 1 calorie per ounce of water. So if you toss back eight glasses of cold water a day, you'll burn about 62 calories. That adds up to 430 calories a week, according to Ellington Darden, Ph.D., author of *A Flat Stomach ASAP.*

# Getting the Most

**Eat for drink.** Drinking isn't the only way to get more water in your diet. Many foods are also very high in moisture. Having soups or stews, for example, can be a big help toward getting your daily water allowance, says Dr. Kaiser. "For even more fluid, add some crunchy vegetables like celery and peppers to these dishes," she says.

**Pick some fruit.** Juicy fruits like watermelons, cantaloupes, oranges, and grapefruits are mostly water, so they're an excellent (and convenient) way to get more water in your diet, Dr. Kaiser says.

**Choose your drinks carefully.** Though juices and decaffeinated tea count toward your daily water total, caffeine-containing drinks like coffee and cola do not. In fact, along with alcohol, caffeinated drinks are diuretics, meaning they pull more water out of your body than they put in. Drinking a glass of water for every caffeine- or alcohol-containing drink will help you break even.

# Wheat

## THE "E" GRAIN

Forget corn, oats, rice, or rye. For Americans wheat is by far the number one grain. The average American, in fact, eats 148 pounds of wheat, in the form of pasta, bread, bagels, and cereals, a year.

One reason that we eat so much wheat is that it's a remarkably versatile grain. It has a light flavor that works well in all kinds of foods, from the flakiest biscuits to the heartiest polentas. And like all grains, wheat is rich in vitamins, minerals, and complex carbohydrates.

But what makes wheat truly special is that it contains one thing that many foods do not: vitamin E. This is important because vitamin E is mainly found in cooking oils such as safflower and canola oils. As a result, getting the Daily Value (DV) of 30 international units of vitamin E can be tricky unless you choose your foods carefully, says Susan Finn, Ph.D., director of nutrition services at Ross Laboratories in Cleveland.

Eating more wheat makes it just a little bit easier. It's worth doing, Dr. Finn adds, because vitamin E may play a direct role both in lowering cholesterol and in preventing it from sticking to artery walls, which can help reduce the risk of heart disease.

### A VITAMIN FOR THE HEART

Every day, the body produces an enormous number of free radicals, which are harmful oxygen molecules that have lost an electron. As a result, these molecules go zipping through the body, grabbing extra electrons wherever they can find them. In the process they damage cholesterol in the bloodstream, making it sticky and more likely to stick to artery walls—the first step in causing heart disease.

Research has shown that eating more wheat can help stop this process from getting started. In a study of 31,000 people, for example, researchers found that those who ate the most whole-wheat bread had a much lower risk of heart disease than those who ate white bread.

Doctors speculate that the vitamin E in wheat causes the liver to produce less cholesterol, says Michael H. Davidson, M.D., president of the Chicago Center for Clinical Research. In one study, for example, people with high cholesterol were given 20 grams (about a quarter-cup) of wheat germ a day for four weeks. (Most of the vitamin E in wheat is concentrated in the germ layer.) Then, for 14 weeks after that, they upped the amount to 30 grams. At the end of the study, researchers found that their cholesterol levels had dropped an average of 7 percent.

Wheat germ is a very concentrated source of vitamin E, with a little less than 2 tablespoons providing 5 international units, about 16 percent of the DV. Oat bran and whole-wheat breads and cereals also contain vitamin E, although in smaller amounts than the germ.

## A FIBER FIND

If you remember the oat bran frenzy of a few years ago, you already know that this grain is prized for its high fiber content. But Mr. Ed's favorite breakfast isn't the only way to get a lot of fiber in your diet. Wheat bran, in fact, contains more than $1^1/_2$ times the fiber of oat bran, and that's good news for your health.

The fiber in wheat, called insoluble fiber, absorbs large amounts of water as it passes through the intestine, causing stools to get larger and heavier. The larger stools pass through the body more quickly—which means that any harmful substances they contain have less time to damage cells in the colon, says Beth Kunkel, R.D., Ph.D., professor of food and nutrition at Clemson University in South Carolina.

When researchers analyzed more than 13 international studies involving more than 15,000 people, they found that those who got the most fiber had a substantially lower risk of developing colon cancer. The researchers estimated that if people would increase the amount of fiber in their diets to 39 grams a day, their risk of colon cancer might drop as much as 31 percent.

One serving of All-Bran cereal, which is made from wheat, has close to 10 grams of fiber. That's almost 40 percent of the DV, all in one bowl. Wheat germ is also a good fiber source, with a little less than 2 tablespoons providing more than 1 gram. Bulgur, whole-wheat pasta, and cracked wheat (which is used to make taboulleh) are other good fiber finds, says Dr. Finn.

# Getting the Most

**Buy it whole.** To get the most vitamin E and fiber from wheat, it's important to buy foods containing wheat germ or whole wheat, which contain the outer, more-nutritious parts of the grain. Once wheat has been processed—when making white bread or "light" cereals, for example—most of the protective ingredients are lost, says Dr. Finn.

**Check the labels.** Some foods that say "whole wheat" on the package contain only a smattering of whole wheat inside. To be sure you're getting the real thing, read the label, says Dr. Finn. When you see "whole wheat" or "whole-wheat flour" at the top of the ingredient list, you know you're making a good choice.

# Yogurt

## THE BENEFITS OF BACTERIA

If someone suggested that you swallow a spoonful of live organisms, you wouldn't do it on a bet. But what if they told you that every spoonful would provide dramatic improvements in your health?

Millions of Americans willingly eat millions of live organisms every day when they open containers of yogurt. Yogurt is positively brimming with bacteria—the live and active cultures that you read about on the label. Research has shown that these "friendly" bacteria can strengthen the immune system and help ulcers heal more quickly. The bacteria also may help prevent recurrent yeast infections, says Eileen Hilton, M.D., an infectious disease specialist at Long Island Jewish Medical Center in New York. And even if you took the bacteria out of yogurt, it would still be a super source of calcium—better, in fact, than a serving of low-fat milk.

### STOPPING THE YEAST BEAST

If you've ever had a yeast infection, you know that you never want to get another one. Eating more yogurt, Dr. Hilton says, may help prevent them from occurring.

Yeast infections occur when a fungus that normally lives in the vagina suddenly multiplies, causing itching, burning, and other uncomfortable symptoms. A study at Long Island Jewish Medical Center suggests that eating live-culture yogurt, especially yogurt containing bacteria called *Lactobacillus acidophilus*, may help keep the fungus under control.

In the study, women who frequently had yeast infections were asked to eat 8 ounces of yogurt a day for six months. At the end of the study, the rate of yeast infections had dropped significantly. The women were so satisfied, in fact, that when researchers asked them to stop eating yogurt, many of them refused to give it up.

The Long Island researchers speculate that eating yogurt helps keep the vagina's natural bacterial environment in balance, making it harder for the yeast fungus to thrive. Additional studies need to be done, Dr. Hilton adds, but in the meantime, women who are trying to prevent yeast infections may want to try eating 1 cup of yogurt a day—the same amount that was used in the study.

It's important, however, to eat yogurt that contains live cultures, Dr. Hilton adds. Yogurt that has been heat-treated doesn't contain bacteria and probably won't be effective. Read the label to find out if your brand has been heat-treated.

## HELP FOR IMMUNITY

You probably remember the television commercials for yogurt that featured hearty, 100-year-old Russians hiking up rocky peaks with energy to spare. The ads were an exaggeration, of course, but yogurt's healthful reputation is not.

The same bacteria in yogurt that help prevent yeast infections can also strengthen the immune system. In one study, for example, researchers at the University of California, Davis, found that people who ate 2 of cups yogurt a day for four months had about four times more gamma interferon, a protein that helps the immune system's white blood cells fight disease, than people who did not eat yogurt. "Gamma interferon is the best mechanism the body has to defend itself against viruses," says Georges Halpern, M.D., Ph.D., professor emeritus in the department of internal medicine at the University of California, who was author of the study.

There's some evidence that yogurt may work against bacterial infections as well. In a laboratory study conducted by researchers at the Netherlands Institute for Dairy Research, animals given yogurt had much lower levels of salmonella bacteria, a common cause of food poisoning, than animals given milk. What's more, the bacteria that did survive had little impact on the animals given yogurt.

## ULCER RELIEF

Since most ulcers are caused by bacteria, the usual treatment is to give large doses of antibiotics. But there's good evidence that eating plenty of live-culture yogurt can keep ulcer-causing bacteria under control, says Patrick Quillin, R.D., Ph.D., vice-president of nutrition for the Cancer Treatment Centers of America.

When you eat yogurt, the beneficial bacteria take up residence inside the digestive tract. Once in place, they begin competing with the harmful bacteria that cause ulcers, Dr. Quillin explains. This makes it more difficult for the ulcer-causing germs to thrive.

In addition, yogurt contains a natural sugar called lactose, which breaks down into lactic acid during digestion. The lactic acid helps restore a healthful environment in the intestine, says Dr. Quillin.

If you have an ulcer, try eating between 1 and 4 cups of yogurt a day, recommends Isadore Rosenfeld, M.D., clinical professor of medicine at New York Hospital–Cornell Medical Center in New York City and author of *Doctor, What Should I Eat?* Just be sure to buy yogurt that says "live and active cultures" on the label.

## CALCIUM WITHOUT PAIN

Even though the large amounts of calcium in low-fat milk make it one of the most healthful foods you can find, many people simply can't drink a lot of it. In fact, doctors estimate that more than 30 million Americans don't have enough of the enzyme (lactase) needed to digest the sugar (lactose) in milk.

Yogurt, however, is an easy-to-digest alternative. Even though yogurt does contain lactose, the live bacteria help the body break it down, so it's less likely to cause discomfort, says Barbara Dixon, R.D., a nutritionist in Baton Rouge, Louisiana, and author of *Good Health for African Americans.* And when it comes to calcium, yogurt is a super source, with 1 cup of plain low-fat yogurt providing 414 milligrams, more than 40 percent of the Daily Value. Compare that to low-fat milk, with just 300 milligrams per serving.

# Getting the Most

**Eat it cold.** Since the bacteria in yogurt can't withstand high heat, it's best to eat your yogurt cold. When you do use yogurt for cooking—when making a sauce, for example—add it when the dish is finished cooking and has been removed from the heat.

**Buy it fresh.** Fresh yogurt contains about 100 million bacteria in a single gram. After a few weeks on the shelf, however, that number quickly dwindles. To get the most of these healing cultures, try to buy yogurt that's less than a week old. Your best bet is to get it from health food stores. Since these stores usually sell a lot of yogurt, you have a much better chance of getting it fresh off the truck.

# Index